D0425900

Health Care Reform Now!

George C. Halvorson

JOSSEY-BASS

Health Care Reform Now!

A Prescription for Change

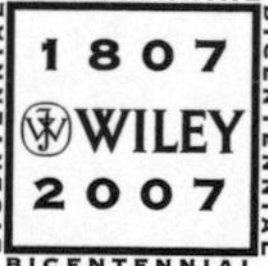

John Wiley & Sons, Inc.

Published by Jossey-Bass
A Wiley Imprint
989 Market Street, San Francisco, CA 94103-1741 www.josseybass.com

Jossey-Bass books and products are available through most bookstores. To contact Jossey-Bass directly call our Customer Care Department within the U.S. at 800-956-7739, outside the U.S. at 317-572-3986, or fax 317-572-4002.

Jossey-Bass also publishes its books in a variety of electronic formats. Some content that appears in print may not be available in electronic books.

Library of Congress Cataloging-in-Publication Data

Halvorson, George C.
Health care reform now! : a prescription for change / George C. Halvorson. — 1st ed.
p. ; cm.
Includes bibliographical references and index.
ISBN 978-0-7879-9752-6 (cloth)
1. Health care reform—United States. 2. Medical economics—United States.
3. Insurance, Health—United States. I. Title.
[DNLM: 1. Health Care Reform—economics—United States. 2. Economics, Medical—organization & administration—United States. 3. Insurance—organization & administration—United States. WA 540 AA1 H118h 2007]
RA395.A3H3449 2007
338.4'33621—dc22

2007011636

Printed in the United States of America
FIRST EDITION
HB Printing 10 9 8 7 6 5 4 3 2 1
PB Printing 10 9 8 7 6 5 4 3 2 1

Contents

This book is dedicated to my four sons and four grandchildren: the reasons we need to make care wonderful and affordable for a very long time ahead.

Acknowledgments

A number of people helped me with this book, offering thoughts, feedback, insight, counsel, and support. I'd like to thank Jay Crosson, M.D., Arthur Southam, M.D., Lon O'Neil, Paul Wallace, M.D., Raymond Baxter, Ph.D., Steve Zatkin, L.L.D., Patricia Lynch, Robert Crane, Diane Lofgren, Lorie Schaible, Nicole Kohleriter, Candice Key, Jennifer Green, Jo Ellen Green Kaiser, and Louise Liang, M.D., for helping me think these issues through. I'd also like to thank George Isham, M.D., for his thought partnership around health care reform. Paul Wallace, M.D., deserves special thanks for his help with Chapter Four, the chapter on chronic disease treatment. He and the Care Management Institute team added value that was beyond the call of duty.

I thank you all.

Introduction

If current rates of health care spending continue, the cost of family health insurance coverage in America will exceed $17,000 per family within four years.[1] Many families will pay over $20,000 per year within five years.[2]

Family health insurance rates in California already exceed the complete per capita income of 147 countries.[3] The cost of family coverage already exceeds the full minimum wage for a single worker in the United States.[4] General Motors now spends more money on health care than it spends on steel.[5] Starbucks spends more on health care than it does on coffee.[6]

We spend more money on health care by far than any other country, and yet more than forty-five million Americans are uninsured at least part of the time each year.[7] To make matters worse, well-documented studies show us that nearly 50 percent of the time American patients are receiving less than adequate, inconsistent, and, too often, unsafe care.[8]

We have reached the point where both health care delivery and health care financing in America need new directions. The old approach isn't technically broken—because it continues to function—but it performs at unacceptable and unaffordable levels in far too many ways for far too many people. Our current approaches to care delivery and health care financing are sadly inadequate for what we need health care to do in this country today.

We don't really have a health care delivery system in this country. We have an expensive plethora of uncoordinated, unlinked, economically segregated, operationally limited microsystems, each performing in ways that too often create suboptimal performance both for the overall health care infrastructure and for individual patients. We have, at best, a nonsystem of care and, truth be told, the current nonsystem of care is inconsistent, massively expensive, sometimes dangerous, operationally inefficient, and dysfunctionally and sometimes perversely incented. Our current approach to financing both care and health care coverage too often leaves us with major operational problems as well as serious ethical issues relative to resource allocation. Our current approach to health care resource consumption can lead to unconscionably inadequate access to quality care for far too many Americans. Those problems are exacerbated for minority Americans. When it comes to racial and ethnic disparities in care and coverage, we very sadly have grown to accept as the status quo in America what should be seen as completely unacceptable differences in care delivery and care outcomes for our various minority populations. Our current nonsystem is expensive, frequently ineffective, and the distribution of care resources is often dangerously and shamefully inequitable.

This is clearly the wrong place to be. I am definitely not the only person who believes that to be true. Far from it. Just about everyone who thinks seriously about American health care today is coming to that same conclusion. It's obviously time for a change—and multiple change agents in our society are increasingly ready to move to a better approach. In my job as CEO of a fairly large health care organization, I've talked to the heads of major unions, senior political leaders, senior community leaders, and the heads of more than a dozen major U.S. corporations. Over the past couple of years, I've talked to industry consultants, to the human resource leaders for a lot of companies, and to senior executives from quite a few leading health care institutions. I've also talked to friends, neighbors, consumers, patients, and various people involved in community activities. Without exception, I hear a call for change. Now. People have lost patience. The time for change truly is upon us.

The problem is—change to what? There isn't a consensus about what we should change to. Everyone knows the problems. No one knows the solution. So we have an incredible tsunami for change building up massive levels of societal energy, with nowhere for that powerful—but currently undirected and unfocused—wave to go.

That's one purpose of this book—to point in one possible direction toward a total package of health care reform that might actually solve major portions of the quality problem, mitigate and significantly improve the cost problem, resolve much of the societal inequity that results from having so many people uninsured, and help solve that full set of economic problems in a way that is uniquely American. Moving to universal coverage has to be part of that solution.

Every Country Takes Its Own Path to Universal Coverage

I've looked at the universal coverage plans of twenty other countries and talked directly to the health ministers of half a dozen to learn how other countries have dealt with those same issues. What I learned was that even though every other industrialized country has achieved universal coverage, they have each taken their own unique path to get there. The Canadian system, British system, and German system are not identical. The approach each country has chosen to get to universal coverage—and much lower overall health care costs than our costs in this country—all fit the specific local logistics and the unique economic and cultural needs, values, belief systems, and characteristics of each country. I have learned that each and every country has designed its own unique version of universal coverage based on the local economic and political characteristics unique and relevant to each country.

I mention that because I believe we need to do the same thing here—evolve to an American system that achieves universal coverage for this country using those specific characteristics of care delivery and financing that are most valued by the American public and the American electorate.

Simply cloning and transplanting Canadian health care is not a viable option. Doing significantly better than Canada is. Stealing a few good ideas from Canada makes a ton of sense. But in the end, if we want to truly succeed, we need our own approach to getting coverage for everyone in America.

A major portion of this book is written to offer a series of facts, data points, observations, and functionally practical suggestions about how we can create a more patient-centered American health care marketplace that offers patients truly well-informed choices, affordable coverage, and an array of fully accountable health care providers competing for patients in the context of value, performance, and cost. We need an American approach that builds effectively and directly on the principles of continuous process improvement to enhance American care delivery while making care more accessible and affordable.

I don't approach these problems from an academic perspective. From a purely functional point of view, I've been directly involved in or worked closely with pretty close to every level and category of health care financing and delivery over the past three decades. Over those years, I've worked in health insurance, health plan management, care system management, and direct care delivery operations. In my current job, I'm the chair and CEO of one of the larger hospital systems in America and the third largest health plan in the country. Over the past three decades, I've worked with the private market, Medicare, Medicaid, and various other governmental programs. I've also had some experience in other countries, starting a health plan in Jamaica quite a few years ago and helping start twenty small health plans in Africa only a few years ago. I'm currently board president for the International Federation of Health Plans—an association of seventy-five independent, operational health plans from twenty-five countries, ranging from Botswana to the United Kingdom to Hong Kong.[9] So I have not limited my thinking about possible approaches and solutions to purely American experiences or purely local thought processes.

The organization I work for in my day job is a special entity. Kaiser Permanente is a vertically integrated organization of medical groups, hospitals, and health plans. We have over 140,000 total employees and involvement in every level of care delivery. Our health plan has nearly nine million members and annual revenue of roughly $35 billion. I love our approach and our model. It truly is a special organization. We bring a lot of health care financing and care delivery functions together under our organizational approach. But I need to recognize here that Kaiser Permanente's vertically integrated organization model and our melded approach to care and coverage are relatively unique within the United States—though there are fairly similar organizational units embedded in the national health systems of several European countries.

Within our vertically integrated organization, we are actively pursuing an aggressive agenda to implement a completely automated medical record system with all care digitized—from scans and X-rays available everywhere through hospital lab test ordering, care delivery best-practice reminders, and direct patient interaction with their medical records. Our goal is to be completely connected, easily accessible, and almost paper-free. It's a relatively unique multibillion dollar system and operational improvement agenda that we are pursuing in large part because of many of the points and perspectives you will read in this book.

This is not, however, a book about us or a book recommending that everyone else become clones of Kaiser Permanente—though I do love our model and believe it offers a wealth of value. So why don't I recommend that everyone else become exactly like us? Because there is no feasible way for the entire country to quickly become a fully vertically integrated system—like Kaiser Permanente—just as there is no feasible way for the United States to completely adopt the Canadian universal coverage system and then move to direct governmental budget control over every single American hospital. There are just too many complications involved in both of those potential ideas for either of them to happen quickly or functionally in this country today. I do believe we would benefit by having more Kaiser Permanente clones in this country, but that is not likely to happen anytime soon, and that's not the point of this book.

So what I advocate in this book is a slightly different model from ours—a model of virtual integration rather than true vertical integration—that I believe can work for everyone else in American health care in a fairly quick time frame.

The model I recommend builds on and emulates some of the best features of a fully integrated approach using computers and care support technology to consistently and systematically improve care delivery and financing across the current American nonsystem of care.

The care delivery approaches, economic incentives, market infrastructure, and universal coverage recommendations proposed by this book are intended to include everyone—involving America's community clinics, our safety net hospitals, and all private and public care delivery systems, ranging from the Mayo Clinics, Geisinger Medical System, and other giant multilevel practices down to the millions of stand-alone independent caregivers who deliver most health care services in this country. The model I am proposing utilizes the best features of the private American health insurance system and incorporates full use of both Medicare and Medicaid infrastructure and financing. It's an American model aimed at building on the best of what America has available right now to deliver and finance care.

This Is the Right Time for Reform

My goal is for this book to be useful to you in thinking clearly with good information about some of these truly complex issues. I do believe it's time to reform American health care, and I believe that if we put in place the right reform agenda, care will be better, more accessible, more universal, and significantly more affordable when we are done.

This is the time. The energy is here now, waiting to be focused. What we need to do at this point is bring everyone—labor, management, consumers, carriers, the uninsured, the underinsured, caregivers, government agencies, patients, and the community together to form a consensus on an approach that can truly get the job done. Then we need to turn that consensus into practical, functional, operational reality as soon as we can get that whole agenda in place.

I hope this book helps in that process. It's intended to be a simple conversation in practical and commonsense terms about some things we need to focus on and some things we need to do to actually reform health in America. *Epidemic of Care* and *Strong Medicine*, two books I wrote earlier, started down this road.[10] This book is the next step on that journey. It's a step toward action. Let me know what you think of the points and ideas that are discussed and proposed. I'd love to hear your reaction and your thoughts.

Be well.

The Author

George C. Halvorson was named chairman and chief executive officer of Kaiser Foundation Health Plan, Inc., and Kaiser Foundation Hospitals, headquartered in Oakland, California, in March 2002. Kaiser Permanente is the nation's largest integrated health plan, serving more than 8.7 million members in nine states and the District of Columbia.

Halvorson has more than thirty years of health care management experience. He was formerly president and CEO of HealthPartners, headquartered in Minneapolis. Prior to joining HealthPartners, he held several senior management positions with Blue Cross and Blue Shield of Minnesota. He was also president of Senior Health Plan and president of Health Accord International, an international HMO management company.

Halvorson serves on a number of boards, including those of America's Health Insurance Plans and the Alliance of Community Health Plans. He is the current president of the Board of Directors of the International Federation of Health Plans, and a member of the Harvard Kennedy School Healthcare Delivery Policy Program, the Commonwealth Fund Commission on a High Performance Health System, and the new Institute of Medicine Task Force on Evidence-Based Medicine. He also serves on the Executive Council of La Clínica, and on the Ambassadors Council to Freedom from

Hunger, an international development organization working in seventeen countries. He is a former board member and trustee of the National Cooperative Business Association.

In addition to *Health Care Reform Now!* Halvorson is the author of other books on health care, including *Epidemic of Care* (2003), *Strong Medicine* (2003), and *Health Care Co-Ops in Uganda: Effectively Launching Micro Health Plans in African Villages* (2006). He is currently writing a new book about racial prejudice around the world. He has written numerous articles on subjects ranging from health information technology to the changing marketplace.

Halvorson has interacted in a number of settings with academics, policymakers, and health industry leaders including the HR Policy Association, the World Bank, the European Health Care Congress, the National Business Group on Health, the Microsoft Annual Health Plan Executive Forum, the National Governors Association, the World Health Care Congress, and a number of universities and colleges. He has served as an advisor to the governments in Great Britain, Jamaica, Uganda, and Russia on issues of health policy and financing.

Health Care Reform Now!

1

A Few Hard but Useful Truths

If we truly want to reform health care in this country, we need to start by addressing four key facts about health care in the United States today. Unless we understand those four facts and deal directly with each one, I believe health care reform, universal health coverage, a consumer-driven health care marketplace based on actual value, and continuous and systematic quality improvement in care delivery will all be unattainable goals.

So what are those four fundamental facts? They are pretty basic, but they need to be clearly stated so we can incorporate them into our thought processes, discussions, and problem-solving approaches. The four key facts are that (1) health care costs are unevenly distributed in America, (2) care linkage deficiencies abound—and can impair or cripple care delivery, (3) economic incentives significantly influence health care, and (4) systems thinking isn't usually on the health care radar screen. Those four realities underpin our current health care dilemma. Dealing directly with each of them will point us toward a practical and achievable health reform solution.

Truth One: Care Costs Are Unevenly Distributed

The first key fact we all need to understand clearly is that health care costs are not distributed evenly across the American population. A very small number of patients spend most of our health care dollars.

Let me make this point in very clear and simple words: any attempt to reform or improve health care expense and cost levels that does not understand and then deal directly with that key cost distribution fact is doomed to fail.

So how skewed are our health care expenses? Very. The specific numbers vary a bit from population to population, but the patterns of spending are the same for every set of people in America.

When we aggregate data for the U.S. population as a whole who have health coverage, 1 percent of the population spends over 35 percent of all health care dollars. Data compiled by our actuaries from various sources indicate that 5 percent of the population spends almost 60 percent. Ten percent spends nearly 70 percent of our care dollars. Our actuaries also calculate that a mere 0.5 percent of the insured population spends nearly 25 percent of all care dollars.[1]

You can see these numbers in Figure 1.1. So the truth is a fairly small number of people spend almost all of our available health care dollars.

On one end of the cost continuum spectrum, a very small number of people spend a very large percentage of our health care dollars. On the other end of that same continuum, there are a lot of people in this country who spend very few health care dollars. Half of the population spends only 3 percent of our health care resources. In dollar terms, the difference between health care spending for those who spend the most and the ones in the bottom 50 percent who spend the least is almost $35,000 per person per year. And 15 percent of our population spends no health care dollars at all in any given year.[2] Zero.

It's hard to reduce costs below zero—so that's obviously not where we should be focusing our attention. Nor should we focus on the folks who spend less than 3 percent of our health care dollars. We need to focus on the big spenders. Thinking strategically and systematically, the key opportunity for us in American health care is obviously to figure out how to have a real impact on the current and future costs of care for those few, very expensive people. Look at Figure 1.1 for some key numbers.

Figure 1.1. Distribution of U.S. Health Care Spending.

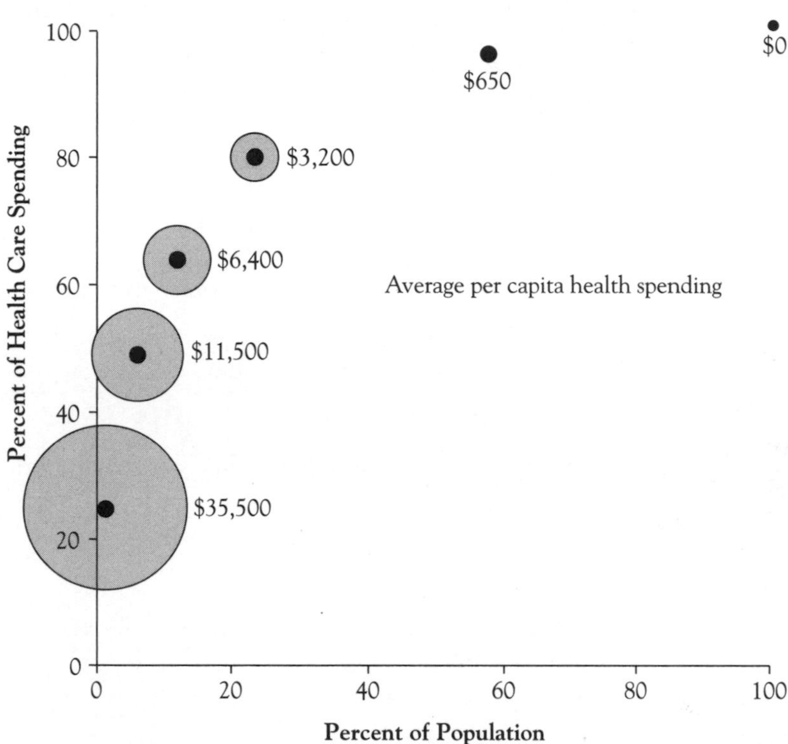

Source: Agency for Healthcare Research and Quality. "Medical Expenditure Panel Survey Statistical Brief #81: Concentration of Health Care Expenditures in the U.S. Civilian Noninstitutionalized Population." May 2005. http://www.meps.ahrq.gov/mepsweb/data_files/publications/st81/stat81.pdf.

Five Chronic Diseases Create the Most Costs

An equally important point of fact that we need to understand and focus on is exactly who spends those dollars. The total medical care costs for people with chronic disease account for more than 70 percent of the nation's health care expenditures.[3] Five basic diseases create the vast majority of American health care expenses, and they are all chronic conditions. Most people do not understand that basic fact of health care economics. Why? Because acute care cases tend to get more attention.

Acute (nonchronic) health conditions tend to get more public attention because each individual acute case can be very visible. Those diseases do not create most health care costs. Pure acute medical conditions like cancer, trauma, infectious diseases, and maternity care do create real expenses, but they are *not* our major cost drivers. Our dollars are overwhelmingly going to people with one or more of these five chronic conditions: diabetes, congestive heart failure, coronary artery disease, asthma, and depression.

That set of facts tells us that we need to think strategically and clearly about those five very expensive conditions if we truly want to impact health care costs in America. We need to learn to think systematically about the care we deliver for each of those diseases and then act systematically to improve the quality, outcomes, consistency, and cost of that care.

Chronic Diseases Progress

For starters, we need to recognize the very useful fact that each of those five very expensive chronic diseases tends to be progressive. They each tend to start with a relatively low level of needed care for each patient. If the patient does not receive proper treatment, his or her condition will worsen until the patient requires major additional amounts of money for his or her care. The expense climbs for each patient over time as his or her health status deteriorates and each person's disease progresses into its full-blown, highly expensive, acute care crisis stages.

Why do we all need to understand that particular fact? Because if we think systematically about that situation, then it becomes obvious pretty quickly that slowing or preventing the progression of each chronic disease from the relatively inexpensive early stage to the incredibly expensive, crisis-laden, and more complex late stage is a huge and obvious opportunity for us all. Successful interventions in the progression of chronic disease have the potential to significantly reduce health care costs and simultaneously improve the quality of life for those chronic care patients. Do the math. If we want to reduce the amount of money we spend on health care, we need to start by recognizing who we are spending it on now, and then we need to improve outcomes and care for those patients so we can reduce the expenses of their care.

This is not just a hope or a dream. Medical science has now progressed to the point where we can effectively intervene in systematic and consistent ways to reduce the complications that drive so many of our health care costs. Any attempt at reforming care delivery or alleviating costs absolutely needs to address these issues directly and take advantage of these opportunities. Interventions are needed. They are possible. They just aren't systematically done in American health care today.

This is a very doable agenda. But it's not how the American health care infrastructure performs now, and this particular cost and quality opportunity is not where most health care reform thinkers currently focus their thinking.

The Impact of Comorbidities

So what else do we need to know about patients with chronic diseases? A key point for each of us to have on our strategic radar screen is the reality and impact of comorbidities. Comorbidities mean that a patient has multiple diseases. It is particularly important to clearly understand that the people getting the most expensive and heaviest levels of care in America today usually have comorbidities—two or more of those five chronic diseases—with an additional acute disease often creating further complex and extremely expensive problems for many of these chronic care patients. See Figures 1.2 and 1.3. Patients with comorbidities generally require the most care, and they often utilize many more caregivers than people with just one disease.[4]

As you will read later in this section, our health care infrastructure does a much worse job of taking care of people with comorbidities

Figure 1.2. Increase in Average Annual Health Care Spending with Comorbidities.

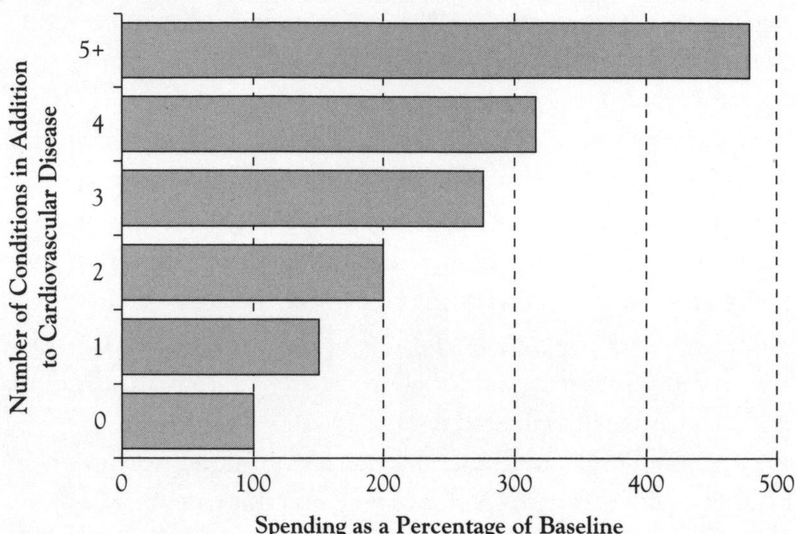

Source: Partnership for Solutions. "Cardiovascular Disease: The Impact of Multiple Chronic Conditions." Baltimore, Md.: Robert Wood Johnson Foundation and Johns Hopkins University, May 2002. http://www.partnershipforsolutions.org/statistics/issue_briefs.html.

than it does of taking care of people with only one disease. In other words, we do least well as an American care infrastructure for the very patients who need care the most.

Those are a couple of key facts about the distribution of health care costs in America that need to be at the foundation of our strategic and operational thinking about care and the costs of care.

Any plan for health care reform that does not deal directly and effectively with those five chronic conditions—and their comorbidities—is probably going to be an exercise in futility—very probably a waste of political, social, and economic energy and resources. Those five conditions are what cause us to spend the bulk of our health care money. It's almost silly to think about health care reform

Figure 1.3. Increase in Average Annual Number of Physician Visits with Comorbidities.

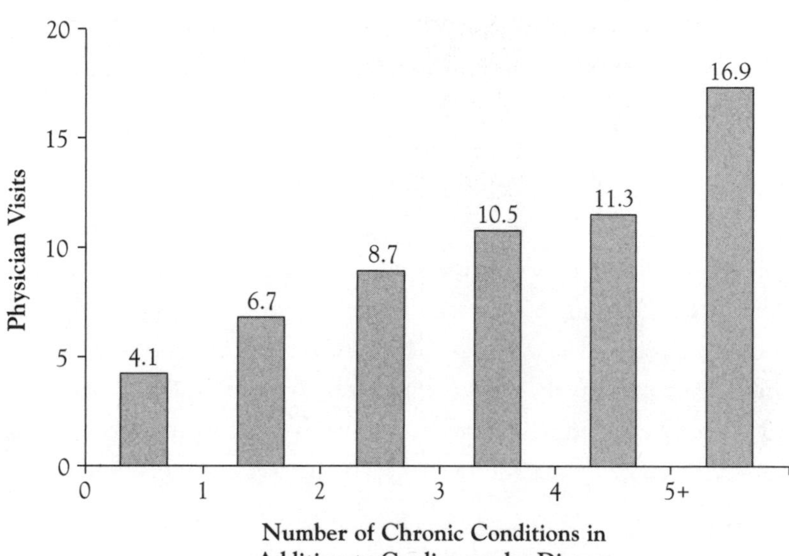

Source: Partnership for Solutions. "Cardiovascular Disease: The Impact of Multiple Chronic Conditions." Baltimore, Md.: Robert Wood Johnson Foundation and Johns Hopkins University, May 2002. http://www.partnershipforsolutions.org/statistics/issue_briefs.html.

that doesn't address each one of these conditions, problems, and opportunities very directly.

Significant Problems with Chronic Disease Care

So how well do we do now in America taking care of those chronic diseases? We don't do well at all.

A wonderful and important study done by the RAND Corporation took a look at the health care of 7,000 Americans, checking every aspect of their care for multiple years. That superb RAND study showed that Americans today receive appropriate care for their complete set of medical conditions barely half of the time[5]—and our care delivery process was particularly inept in providing care to people with those five chronic diseases.

That's not the only research that has resulted in that finding. John Wennberg's wonderful work at Dartmouth Medical School[6] (see Figure 1.4) and a body of excellent work done by the prestigious Institute of Medicine (IOM)[7] both point us to equally dramatic and troubling conclusions. According to the IOM, there is a vast "chasm" between the care we know people should get and the care that patients in America actually receive. The IOM wrote a book titled *Crossing the Quality Chasm* that should be required reading for anyone advocating health care reform in America. [8] It's a brilliant piece of work. Easy to read. Well argued. Well documented. Absolutely clear in its message. If you haven't read it, please get a copy. The introduction alone is worth the price of the book.

Box 1.1. The Institute of Medicine on the State of U.S. Health Care.

Crossing the Quality Chasm makes the point that the current state of the health care delivery system is mismatched to the needs of U.S. citizens, particularly those with chronic disease. The Institute of Medicine (IOM) concluded that bringing state-of-the-art care to Americans in every community requires a sweeping redesign of the entire health care system for patients to receive care that is safer, more reliable, more responsive to their needs, more integrated, and more available, and for patients to count on receiving the full array of preventive, acute, and chronic services that are likely to prove beneficial. As a follow-up to this report, seventeen priority areas for transforming health care were identified. These include diabetes, coronary heart failure and coronary artery disease, asthma, and major depression.

Figure 1.4. Regional Differences in the Rate of Cardiac Bypass Surgery.

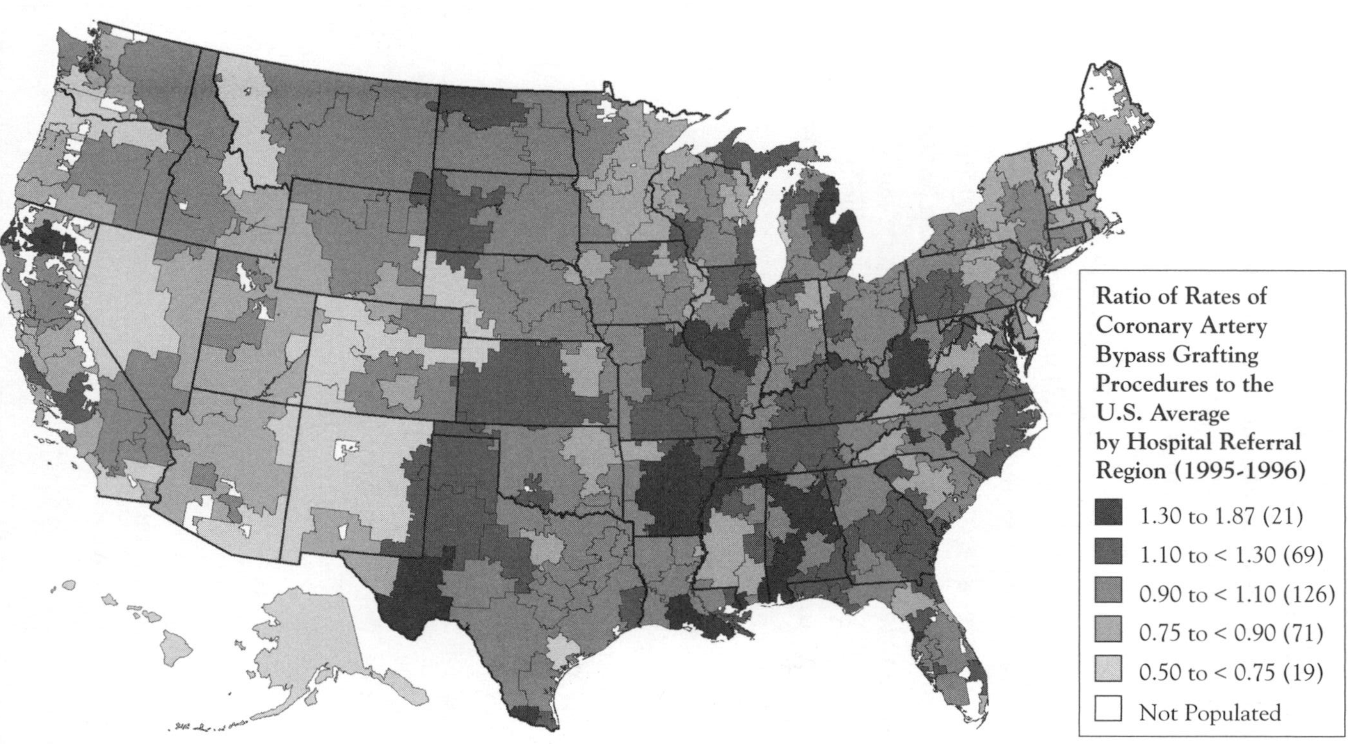

Source: J. E. Wennberg and M. M. Cooper (eds.). "The Quality of Medical Care in the United States: A Report on the Medicare Program." *The Dartmouth Atlas of Health Care 1999*. Chicago, Ill.: Health Forum.

So, back to the first hard truth—we have a very small number of patients running up huge bills for care, those patients tend to suffer from chronic diseases, and we as a nation do a demonstrably inadequate job of providing the specific care those expensive patients need. So what are those chronic diseases?

Diabetes, Congestive Heart Failure, Coronary Artery Disease, Asthma, and Depression

Those five chronic diseases are diabetes, congestive heart failure, coronary artery disease, asthma, and depression. Hypertension is also extremely relevant because it is an underlying health condition that leads to heart failures and exacerbates the complications of diabetes. Those are the big-ticket items—the conditions that create most of our care costs. Following behind those chronic conditions—and—ranked also by expense—are several acute care health conditions, with trauma, cancer, maternity care, and various kinds of bone and joint care leading the cost parade. Cancer, in total, runs about 5 percent of the total U.S. health care dollar.[9] Maternity care runs at roughly 4 percent.[10] Bone and joint care runs just under 2 percent.[11]

I mention those additional less expensive acute care conditions because in a $2 trillion health care economy, 4 percent and 5 percent are still a lot of money. I mention them as well because we also have great opportunities for care improvement for each of these conditions. Too many patients in each of these categories of care also currently suffer from inconsistent, inadequate, and uncoordinated care. How well do we do on maternity care? We rank thirty-fifth in the world in infant mortality,[12] a number that should horrify us as a nation because we spend twice as much money per capita on health care as any nation in the world and, by world performance standards, we do not get what we pay for.[13] There are statistics later in this book about our sometimes dangerous inconsistencies in providing cancer care, orthopedic surgeries and joint care, and maternity care. We have a lot of opportunity to significantly improve care in each of those key acute areas as well.

But that's later in the book. For now, we need to be clear about that first hard truth: a small number of people run up most of the huge health care bill faced by this country. We know exactly who they are. We know from good and credible experience and research that we are not doing a great job on their care. For example, we know from good and credible experience and research that we could cut the complications of people with diabetes by up to 90 percent with best care and involved patients.[14] Other conditions offer similar opportunities. We know that we can cut second heart attacks by over 40 percent[15]—and we know that we could cut school and work days lost because of asthma by nearly 90 percent[16]—and yet we choose as a society and as a national care environment not to systematically and strategically figure out the best ways of going down those clearly available and extremely useful care improvement paths.

As you will read in this book, that is a huge mistake—one we need to correct.

So that's fact one. A small number of people create the vast majority of our health care costs, and we could be doing a much better job of taking care of those people.

The Second Hard Truth: Care Linkage Deficiencies Abound

The second hard truth we all need to face is that our actual frontline care delivery process in this country is weakened, shortchanged, undermined, and sometimes crippled by pervasive care linkage deficiencies. Trained system thinkers from other industries who study how we actually logistically and operationally deliver care in this country quickly note the constant and almost unconscionable gaps that exist related to both the connectivity and coordination between various American caregivers.

A patient with two diseases typically has two doctors—two independent caregivers, each specializing in their particular disease. A patient with three comorbidities typically will have at least three doctors, each representing one of the three separate specialties.

Why is this a problem? Isn't it good that we can offer patients a range of specialists? It is. The problem is that we have no system in place to coordinate the care given by these different doctors.

The Problem with Paper Records

Three doctors means three separate, nonelectronic medical records—multiple pieces of paper about each patient, with each piece of paper stored in separate paper files and each physician's separate record by definition incomplete, noting in relevant detail only the care delivered by that particular doctor for that particular disease in that particular place.

Record keeping for American health care is almost always stored by doctor, not by patient—flawed as that model obviously is from the perspective of overall good and systematic patient-focused care. For patients trying to get a clear sense of their own medical status, having multiple pieces of paper records in multiple sites can be a logistical nightmare. Care records also tend not to follow when the patient moves from one area to another.

For example, a child treated for asthma in San Diego can move to El Paso and, almost without exception, none of the needed care information will follow for the vast majority of patients who move or change caregiver.

Records of care received during an emergency room visit are almost always unavailable during follow-up care with the patient's primary care physician. Needed information from the primary care physician may not be available during a visit to a specialist.[17]

Care Silos

The paper files that people depend on for care information are only part of the problem. Typically, the doctors for a given patient with comorbidities seldom communicate with each other, and the total care for each patient is almost always functionally delivered in care silos, not care systems. Care isn't coordinated, and the important information about the care actually delivered to each patient generally stays with the doctor, not the patient. Patients with cancer and diabetes typically experience no connectivity between their ophthalmologist and their oncologist, even though both are prescribing medications. Those files stay locked in separate buildings and are often not coordinated in any way.

Those care linkage deficiencies (CLDs) cause problems at multiple levels. Doctors are reliant on information. Medicine is an information-driven profession. Doctors who practice without complete information about a given patient are handicapped. Sometimes dangerously handicapped. Studies show that CLDs are known to contribute to unnecessary hospitalizations.[18]

The extent to which care linkages are impaired is often painfully visible to the patient and his or her loved ones when a patient has a serious disease. Anyone who has tried to help an older parent with care needs in any kind of care crisis knows exactly what I'm writing about. If you fly into another town to figure out what level of total care your parents are—and have been—receiving, it's often almost impossible to get the information you want or need. Each relevant caregiver is generally separate and siloed, and treatment coordination between caregivers is extremely rare, rather than the rule or expectation.

Since the most expensive patients that I referred to in the first hard truth tend to have comorbidities, any care delivery approach that doesn't have well-executed coordination built into the overall system is inherently and inevitably going to produce an inferior outcome a very high percentage of the time.

Disincentive to Change

The current constant gaps in systematization create problems, inconveniences, and even tragedies for patients. They add significantly to total health care costs. They also create a complete inability for society overall or for various payers or purchasers of care to create any sense of caregiver and care system accountability or to create effective caregiver and care system performance incentives or rewards.

A fact that some patients are beginning to realize and resent is that most caregivers in this country are making almost no attempts to improve that care linkage deficiency situation. The functional CLD problem is almost completely ignored by the vast majority of caregivers.[19] It's simply not a problem that most caregivers spend any real time trying to correct. Care delivery practitioners usually hold the overall care infrastructure to an incredibly low standard when it comes to the creation and existence of a network or system of adequate communication processes focused on each patient.

If questioned about CLDs, caregivers may acknowledge the generic issue, but then even the best intentioned unlinked caregivers typically shrug in frustration and say, "That's just the way it is. That's how care in America works." Expectations about CLDs are very low. Amazingly low. Anyone trained in formal systems thinking or process improvement methodology who looks at those dysfunctional, unconnected system elements is horrified at how low those caregiver expectations now actually are about linkages between caregivers.

We can and should do a lot better. Even in the world of unlinked solo practice caregivers.

I'll return to those points later. For now, the second major fact we all need to recognize as we try to figure out how to truly reform health care in America is that our current health care delivery process is overrun with significant care linkage deficiencies, and we will not be able to deliver optimal care until adequate, consistent, and dependable care linkages are created and made real for each patient.

There are a number of ways to achieve that goal. I'll cover a couple of approaches later in the book. But we can only start on a solution once we recognize the second hard truth: a multiplicity of care linkage deficiencies that we either tend to accept or ignore as both purchasers and providers of care currently keep us from delivering optimal and efficient care to our most expensive patients.

The result is both lower quality care and higher cost.

The Third Hard Truth: Economic Incentives Significantly Influence Health Care

The third major fact that we all need to be very aware of as we try to reform American health care is that market forces and economic incentives absolutely do work to influence care. The hard truth, however, is that up to now we have almost always used very perverse and frequently counterproductive financial economic incentives for American caregivers.

I've actually had quite a few people ask me why market forces don't seem to have any impact on American health care. People say, "Financial incentives work in every other area of the economy—why is health care exempt from them?" That's an inaccurate diagnosis of the situation. Market forces and economic incentives do work in health care, but the truth is, we haven't designed those incentives very well at this point. So the incentives we use now too often give us unfortunate outcomes. We need to recognize that our caregivers are in fact fully responsive to the specific economic incentives that exist now and that providers of care are actually giving us today exactly what our current economic incentives reward.

Market Incentives Work

Incentives absolutely do work. They work in every other area of the economy and they work in health care. The economic theory on that point is completely valid and well proven.[20] Health care is just like every other economic system. In every industry, market incentives influence and shape the production of goods and services. What does that mean in practical terms? It means that market forces sculpt and screen both products and services. No industry produces goods that customers won't buy. Buying is the key. Every industry produces exactly what the customers actually pay for. Buyers are the final and absolute test. Economic units—businesses—produce what buyers buy, and economic units fail and go out of business if the buyers won't buy what they produce. It's actually a pretty clear, utterly ruthless, and completely rigorous screening process for both products and services.

Anyone who wants to apply market forces more constructively to health care needs to understand that basic truth about how market forces actively work. Customers are the key. Products without customers do not survive. Products with customers thrive. Business units that produce what the customers actually buy have both revenue and economic sustenance. Business units with no revenue are gone quickly. Business units all respond to the customer. You basically get what you pay for, and you survive as an economic unit only if you get paid.

If everyone wants to buy cell phones, a lot of economic units figure out how to produce and sell cell phones. Demand for a product structures what people produce. If you want to know why so many companies produce cell phones today, follow the money. Production follows payment.

So what do we actually pay for in health care today? These are the bare facts: we have over nine thousand billing codes for individual health care procedures, services, and separate units of care.[21] There is not one single billing code for patient improvement. There is also not one single billing code for a cure. Providers have a huge economic incentive to do a lot of procedures. They have no economic incentive to actually make us better. The economic incentive score is 9,000 to zero—process versus results. Results get zero.

So what does the largest health care economy in the world produce? Cures? No. Cures aren't a billable event. Systematic health improvement? No. Health improvement is also not a billable event. No one buys it, so no one sells it. Procedures are, however, easily billable—so our caregivers produce huge numbers of procedures. We generally pay very well for procedures in this country. In response, caregivers produce constantly expanding volumes of individual units of care. Our caregivers sell procedures one by one, and caregivers get paid for doing each procedure—with no portion of that pay ever based on the actual results or success of that procedure. So the economic focus of caregivers is, of course, on individual, billable services. We can't blame providers for having that focus. That's the way providers get paid. So of course, providers focus on the specific pieces of work that actually create payment. That provider focus on billable events needs to be there or providers will not survive in today's health care economy as economic units.

Changing the Incentives

When we stop to think about what we really want to buy in health care, what is it? I suspect health improvement and cures would be pretty high on the list. But sadly, in the current American health care economic model, there is absolutely no systematic billable event or opportunity for caregivers to benefit financially from improving patient outcomes. There is no efficiency payment, no success payment, and no economic reward for improving overall health.

There is also no overall caregiver financial agenda built around any real economic gains that might be earned by a caregiver for achieving very measurable process-based quality improvement goals like reducing the number of acute asthma attacks or shrinking the numbers of expensive care site crisis use by 50 to 90 percent for a given population or for a given disease. Some pay-for-performance programs are being piloted to look at rewarding some levels of performance, process, and results. That's a good thing. But so far, the actual pay-for-performance process at this point is tiny and very experimental.[22]

Take asthma—one of the five chronic diseases—as an example. No one pays providers to reduce either the level or the volume of asthma crisis. Providers are, however, paid a lot of money to take care of an asthma patient who is in a crisis. Hospitals, in fact, make very nice profits off each asthma patient in a crisis who is admitted to the hospital. Hospitals make absolutely no money from an educated, enlightened, and personally empowered asthma patient who recognizes his or her symptoms at an early stage and then takes the steps necessary to avoid an emergency room visit or a hospitalization.

So, whether you are an academic, philosophical, theoretical, or even professional believer in market forces, the question is the same—do you really think the best reward system is to pay providers a lot of money when patients move from good health to bad health—to pay real money only for an expensive, painful, acute asthma crisis—or would it make some economic sense to pay providers well in some viable way for preventing those expensive and extremely unpleasant crises?

Keep in mind what American health care rewards now. This is an extremely important point for us all to recognize. We pay well now for the crisis. An asthma crisis can be a very lucrative event. But preventing that same crisis creates no billable event. And today we are in the middle of a national asthma crisis—an explosion in the number of people having their own individual asthma crisis. In one study, asthma was the third most frequent cause of avoidable hospitalizations.[23] That problem is happening not because caregivers create that crisis—but in part because caregivers have no market-based incentive or revenue stream to use to systematically and proactively intervene to prevent that crisis. No one disputes the fact that we could significantly alleviate this national asthma crisis by treating asthma in a systemic way.

That question of how to pay for care seems to be a lot harder for many people to answer than it should be. It has been complicated for buyers by the fact that it has seemed counterintuitive to believe it is better to somehow pay moderately well for a second heart attack that will never happen rather than to pay very well for a second heart attack that will in fact happen. Until now, the decision has been to pay only for problems after they happen—not to incent the processes or approaches that measurably and effectively prevent those expensive problems from happening at all.

To be fair to the purchasers of care, that resistance to thinking differently about how to pay for care delivery has not been limited to buyers. Providers of care also have tended to oppose any change in the current set of incentives. Just about everyone in the American provider infrastructure is used to the current payment approach.

It's how the care infrastructure gets its money. Fee-for-service payments are easy to calculate. The business model decisions for fee-for-service American providers are not very complex: "I'll perform a defined service; you pay me a defined fee." Many care providers actually love to be paid solely on a piecework basis. The business models of America's massive infrastructure of fee-for-service care providers are now built entirely around piecework care—growing volumes of piecework care. Those business models often are very lucrative for the caregivers.

So a lot of American care providers directly disparage, discourage, and even resist any significant reform efforts relative to health care purchasing or payment approaches. "Fee-for-service medicine is the only way to guarantee quality," they say. "Quality suffers as soon as fee-for-service payments disappear. "

If there's actually a serious quality-of-care guarantee connected in some way to fee-for-service health care, someone in America should be cashing in right now on that guarantee clause, because that particular product value promise has clearly failed. RAND, the IOM, and Wennberg have all proven that supposed fee-for-service linked quality guarantee to be fraudulent.

We all like to think of our caregivers as good people—trying very hard to do the right thing. That is, I believe, actually very true. Our care providers are good people, all trying to do the right thing—but a bit more specifically, everyone is doing the "billable right thing." If it isn't billable, it isn't happening. Successfully preventing a health care crisis is not billable. Care linkages are not billable. So care linkages do not happen.

In a fee-for-service health care world, care linkages almost never exist. But, as I noted earlier, it's pretty hard to simply blame the providers for that reality. No one pays for care linkages. Patients do need them, but no one pays for them. So nobody creates them. Providers can't afford to do work they don't get paid for. That's just practical economic reality. Its also economic common sense. Independent caregivers could literally not survive as economic units if they spent their time doing nonbillable things. Income, revenue, and the economic survival of caregivers all result exclusively from doing billable things. Economic incentives determine both what gets done and what doesn't get done.

My major point here is that health care has already proven that it responds with a passion to existing market forces. Our health care infrastructure has grown to be the biggest in the world, due entirely to the market forces and market rewards we now use. We can see the consequences of the current reward system everywhere we look. We pay specialists more than primary care doctors, so we have very few doctors going into primary care. We pay a lot for diagnostic imaging, so the bills for imaging equipment are growing faster than anything else in health care.[24] The good news is that the new scanning equipment can do wonderful work diagnosing disease. Some of the images are almost magical miracles of technology that directly benefit patients. So I am not generically critical of those procedures. The challenge is that the financial incentives to use those marvelous but expensive machines are not directly linked to their actual value.

Market forces work in health care. The problem has been that the market forces used have been badly flawed. We are creating incentives for some things we really should not incent. And the response to those incentives on the part of the provider community, not surprisingly, has been equally flawed. Completely logical. Entirely understandable. Economically practical. But flawed.

Some people try to refute that point by saying, "At least we get a lot of care with our current set of incentives." That is true. But more care is not necessarily better care. Read the studies by John Wennberg at Dartmouth Medical School on the relationship between high costs, high frequency for care, and low care quality, and you can see pretty clearly how flawed the current economic model is.[25] The Dartmouth database has shown us clearly that the highest-cost communities with the highest level of physician encounters per patient often were the communities with the lowest measurable quality of care. Market forces in those communities created high volumes of services, not better care. Inappropriate levels of care can be dangerous and can damage quality of life for patients. More is not better. What is better? Right care. Right care is far better than just more care. We need to incent best care and right care, not more care.

This book will propose that buyers support and use an alternative market incentive approach and a different market model. For now, the fact I want to point out is that market forces do work to influence care. We see that every day. We need to create market incentives that produce better care, not just more care or inconsistent, dangerous, and inadequate care.

The Fourth Hard Truth: Systems Thinking Is Almost Never on the Health Care Radar Screen

The fourth major foundational fact we all need to look at very carefully and understand very well if we want to functionally reform care delivery in this country is one that is not at all obvious to people outside of care delivery. It may in fact be the single biggest current misperception and misunderstanding about health care delivery that exists on the part of people who are not caregivers.

People believe health care in this country is an actual system with systemic processes fully in place. People tend to believe that when a new medical science learning, insight, treatment, or technology is developed, there is some in-place process today that will get that new science effectively to their personal caregiver. People tend to believe that when their personal doctor recommends a treatment, it's done with a clear sense of what the probable statistical outcomes of that treatment are. People believe that health care operates every day in the context of a living, interactive, up-to-date database that constantly compares one set of treatments to another relative to their likely success levels, with caregivers learning regularly what the most current comparative success levels are. People believe that a lot of systems thinking and data sharing happens in health care. Patients have a high level of comfort that their own personal caregivers and care infrastructure are part of a huge systematic care improvement process.

The truth is there is an almost total lack of systems thinking in health care. Health care is delivered one unit at a time. That's what the market incents. That's where the focus is now. Thinking tends to be focused almost exclusively on those single care units—those individual procedures. Relative outcomes of various care approaches are almost never tracked or measured. Outcomes measurement at any level is on almost no one's radar screen. Comparative and concurrent performance data are not part of the American health care culture—nor typically are performance measurements part of the professional mind-set for individual fee-for-service caregivers at any level, unless those measurements have been somehow externally imposed.

Some measurement happens, but usually only because someone external insisted on the measurement. When regulators, buyers, or credentialing processes very literally require or demand that something be measured, measurement happens.[26] Outside of those infrequent external requirements, measurement is rare. I hate to be so brutally frank, but health care as an overall infrastructure and as provider entities or individual providers of care measures almost nothing when judged by the normal standards of performance tracking that exist for any category of systematic quality improvement processes used by other major industries. Few measurements are taken. And even when those few measurements are done in health care, they generally aren't compared with each other or used in any systematic way for quality improvement processes.

As I noted earlier, the very few aggregate measures that do exist now tend to have been externally imposed by buyers or regulators, and the actual measurement of data in those areas tends to stop at the lowest possible level needed to satisfy the very specific, bare bones, bare minimum levels mandated in each case by the external reporting environment.

Health Care Needs Data

Why is this lack of measurement a problem that we need to understand if we want to reform health care? Reform takes data. Accountability takes data. Real competition takes data. Data is the key. Health care lacks data.

In other industries, data is golden. Data is the mother's milk of systems improvement. Data is the tool that lets hard-working systems and process engineers actually improve processes and outcomes. Data is treasured. Data use is a skill and a science.

In health care, pure scientific data is absolutely and unquestionably respected. Not always used consistently, or even known, but deeply respected. The culture of health care deeply respects, honors, and values good science. But hard as it is to understand, when it comes to operational, functional, process-based data, the culture of health care is very different. Operational data is not particularly respected. Data is not sought after, either. Operational data is in fact just about nonexistent in health care. That type of data isn't valued and the lack of data isn't even noticed or missed.

So the hard truth is having comparative performance data about various aspects of care improvement and care efficiency is not regarded as a potential gold mine for process improvement by caregivers. Performance reporting that actually exists about either processes or outcomes is almost always regarded in the current culture of American health care as an onerous, externally imposed burden, extraneous and irrelevant to the actual business and profession of care delivery.

In any other industry, the specific financial and operational data I mentioned at the beginning of this chapter would be highly valued and broadly utilized information. In another industry, the simple fact that 1 percent of customers use over 35 percent of all organizational resources, for example—that would be the focal point for highly energized thinking and would result in extensive, well-engineered performance improvement efforts. Yet in health care circles, those extremely important numbers are ignored. Simply and literally ignored. Almost no one in health care operations looks at those amazing numbers and says, "There must be something we can consistently, effectively, and systematically do to keep the people with those chronic conditions from getting to that most unaffordable and costly 1 percent status."

Go to any health care conference and try to find anyone who delivers care for a living even talking about those incredibly important numbers. A few concerned people—economists, actuaries, and some enlightened buyers—are beginning to point out those numbers. They are generally getting little or no real-world support for their efforts. I've pointed those numbers out myself in speeches and prior books and articles.[27] The actual data and statistics I've cited are sometimes quoted, but pretty much never acted upon by anyone in health care. Process numbers are extremely rare. Outcomes numbers are even more rare. And almost no one in health care is attempting to set up a process where those kinds of numbers are relevant to decision making at any practical level. That's a major challenge to health care reform. It's hard to fix a system when its basic operations are not built around a numbers-driven thought process—and when very few caregivers even know what the most relevant numbers are.

To be fair, there are some exceptions. A few large multispecialty medical groups like the Mayo Clinic, Intermountain Healthcare, HealthPartners, the Veteran's Administration, and our own Kaiser Permanente physician groups are doing some powerful and effective data-supported process improvement work.[28] But those few megamedical groups—large as they are—make up a very small percentage of the total health care delivery infrastructure of this country. Less than 4 percent of all U.S. physicians work in practices with fifty or more other physicians.[29] For the rest of the caregivers in this country, those kinds of numbers generally drive no operational or strategic analysis and no behavior change. They are interesting—but not inspirational.

The hard fact we need to recognize in thinking about the health care reform agenda we need for this country is that systems thinking is simply not part of the current health care agenda for most caregivers. Systems thinking is not a tool used today on a regular basis by care leaders to transform and improve care delivery. It isn't even discussed as an option in most settings. Data flows are deeply valued everywhere in every non–health care work setting where systematic thinking is done. But they are not usually valued in health care.

Disincentives for Systems Thinking

So why is systems level analytical thinking so rare in health care?

The point here is not to blame the caregivers. Look again to the dollars. The answer is in the economics. What do we incent and what do we reward? Do we reward caregivers for the results of the same kinds of analytic thinking that create economic wins for other industries? Not very often. In fact, usually the opposite economic impact occurs. The payment system itself far too often directly penalizes systems-based efficiency when it actually happens.

When the Mayo Clinic, Park Nicollet Health Services, and HealthPartners Medical Group—a team I was proud to be part of—set up the Institute for Clinical Systems Improvement (ICSI) in Minnesota, our aim was to have the best and brightest caregivers in Minnesota figure out best practices for various types of care. One of the first conditions we looked at through ICSI was simple cystitis—urinary tract infections in women. The medical science identified the best tests, best drugs, best dosages, best processes, and so on to treat cystitis. Then the ICSI team checked to see how many cases were currently treated in Minnesota using that best approach. Roughly 12 percent were. That meant 88 percent were not. So an intensive campaign began to educate participating ICSI member physicians on the best approach to care for women with that specific health problem. What happened? Real improvement. The number of cases treated using the best approach increased by 500 percent within a year—to over 60 percent.[30]

In the world of health care, that was a big win for systems thinking. It used systems thinking to make care better and more efficient. But there was a problem. A serious problem. An unintended glitch.

Patients definitely received better care. But it turned out better care actually produced less revenue for the caregivers by quite a bit. Cost of care went down by 35 percent, more than a third.[31] Getting care right the first time was generally cheaper for the patient than getting it wrong initially and having the caregiver re-treat the patient and then bill for another round of care . . . continuing to treat the patient until a future treatment finally worked. Rework had actually been fairly profitable, when only 12 percent of the doctors were using the best approach. Rework generated a lot of caregiver revenue. So did unnecessary office visits—visits that could be eliminated by patient-focused reengineered care delivery.

So what happened? Think about the model from an economic perspective. The care was better. Revenue was worse.

ICSI doctors took the high road and did the right and honorable thing. ICSI doctors stayed at a higher level of compliance with best care. The results were publicized. And the process never caught on anywhere else in America. No one else wants to lose 35 percent of their billable revenue for their patients. Providers do not see losing 35 percent of their revenue as an economic reward. The current American payment approach directly and immediately penalized the providers who provided best care for those patients. Care was better, but using a systematic approach to reengineer care in favor of better patient health and much better overall care system efficiency hurt individual doctors financially.

The prestigious Virginia Mason Medical Group just made a presentation on a similar program to the MEDPAC Commission in Washington, DC.[32] They applied best practice protocols to the use of imaging services for certain patients. The number of scans that were determined to be medically needed dropped significantly. That was the good news. The bad news was that the medical group revenue from the scans for Virginia Mason also dropped significantly.[33]

The reward for doing good was not to do well—it was to be financially penalized.

The same drop in overall care system revenue happens when the care delivery infrastructure cuts the rate of heart attacks or asthma crises. Revenue drops. No one is rewarded. Caregivers are financially penalized. Incentives to create efficiency do not now exist. Disincentives abound. Guess what happens? Inefficiency rules. That kind of economic result obviously doesn't stimulate or encourage systematic thinking or behavior. It definitely does not create an incentive to gather data that can be used in a systematic way to continually reengineer the process of care delivery.

One of my favorite process improvement stories in health care concerns dental decay. A bright process analyst, patient advocate, and systems thinker many years ago looked at the total process of tooth decay and said, "If we could just intervene very early in the decay process and seal each person's teeth with something that would physically protect each tooth from decay-causing organisms, we could probably make a huge impact on the total amount of dental work each patient needed."

That experiment was done. It worked. Teeth were sealed with a special plastic sealant that covered up the tiny cracks where cavities start. The clinical result was almost a 90 percent reduction in both tooth decay and a significant reduction in the number of dental fillings needed.[34] My own kids had their teeth sealed, and they have had no need for fillings, in either their baby or adult teeth. None. They literally don't know what a dental drill feels like. I very much envy them. They've had their teeth cleaned, but never drilled. Sealants are a clear and basic application of good science and well-thought-out process improvement thinking to care delivery.

So do all dentists in America now seal everyone's teeth? Not all. Less than a third of children have at least one sealant.[35] A cynic might note that any time a dentist seals a tooth, the likelihood of billings for future repair work for that tooth drops off precipitously.

That's a problem for dentists. Dental fillings have been the biggest source of direct revenue for dentists for a very long time.

Prepaid dental plans—organized dental providers who get paid a fixed amount of money for all needed dental care—seal teeth enthusiastically, because those dental plans have a strong economic incentive to avoid future dental costs. Drilling teeth is an expense for prepaid dentists—not a revenue opportunity. By contrast, most fee-for-service dentists seal teeth less enthusiastically, if at all, because those independent business units don't necessarily want to eliminate future revenue.

The bottom line is that dentists who benefit through prepayment approaches for avoiding future cavities seal teeth all the time in very systematic ways. The financial incentive under prepayment to seal those teeth is clear. Incentives do work in health care. So does systems thinking. They each work best when they are carefully linked and aligned.

Systems Thinking, Data, and Doctor Autonomy

So how do we get health care to start thinking systematically? To begin the process, we need data. We need a database that will give us the framework for tracking, monitoring, and comparing performance in key areas of care—like care of people with asthma or diabetes—where we know that the real-world opportunities for fewer crises and fewer complications are huge.

We also need buyers who care about that performance data and then reward the right kind of provider performance. Buyers are the key. Products without buyers don't exist. As noted earlier, products with buyers thrive. We need buyers to create and support market forces to incent best care. We need market forces that reward America's doctors for providing the right care to women with simple cystitis—rather than continuing to use market systems that financially penalize doctors for that same right care. We need the same kinds of thinking that cause prepaid dentists to seal teeth to apply to doctors and care systems who take care of congestive heart failure patients and coronary heart disease patients. We need systems thinking applied to the care of our patients with depression, charting out the right interventions, the right treatments, the right prescriptions, the right tracking, and the right follow-up. Non–systems thinking will just get us to where we are now—the most expensive care delivery economy in the world, with marginal and unmeasured outcomes and over 45 million uninsured people.

I'm not suggesting that we want, need, or should create a marketplace where physicians should be forced into "rules-based" medicine. That would be bad. It is a very good thing for each physician to have professional autonomy in taking care of each patient. We all want and need our personal caregivers to have that kind of autonomy. The doctor-patient relationship is a very special and valuable interaction that should have particular protection as we move forward to reform health care. We should all want our physicians, as professionals and as caring human beings, to be cocaptains of a special and unique one-to-one care relationship, working in full partnership with each of us as individual patients.

When I see my doctor for my own coronary artery disease or for the bone spur in my left shoulder or for my damaged knees from high school football, I want my doctor to have me as his or her primary focus. I want my doctor to be professionally and ethically accountable to me as his or her patient. I want my physician's best professional thinking and best care, unfettered by hierarchies or rules imposed outside the exam room. I also want each of my caregivers to be fully aware of the best medical science relevant to my situation, and I would like to know that my caregivers are part of a competent and interacting physician team and that the medical team is making sure all team members are delivering solid care. I want to know that the care I receive is the right care for my condition and that my doctor and I can make decisions together about that care. I do not want "rules-based" medicine. I do want accountable care.

Right now, for most of health care, there are no aggregate measures of care performance. There is no aggregate or solo accountability for care outcomes. There is no aggregate reward system for improving population health. And there is little or no aggregate systems thinking about how to improve the actual delivery of care.

At the individual physician level, there is almost no tracking of key process and outcome measures in highly relevant ways. No one measures in any consistent way how many patients from a given prostate surgeon become impotent or incontinent. Those numbers vary. Without measurement, our process of physician selection by individual patients is a matter of faith, not information. We can do a lot better. We need systems thinking used for key individual performance arenas as well.

To be very clear, our problem is not that caregivers are consciously and deliberately rejecting systems thinking opportunities. Without data, those opportunities simply do not exist. It's also not the case that there was a specific time when process thinking in health care was ever rejected. Systems thinking typically isn't rejected in health care. It simply hadn't even been considered. Systems thinking opportunities just plain never come up in most health care settings. Without data, systems thinking is not even on the table to be rejected. Typically, in American care settings there are no current data, no comparative data, and no perceived need for data. There are no performance comparisons, and no perceived need for data comparisons.

Should we really want comparative data? Think of that question as a patient yourself. Imagine that you have just been diagnosed with cancer. A potentially terminal cancer. If you hear, as a patient, that over the past decade, one oncology group had a 90 percent five-year survival rate for Stage IA breast cancer, and another group down the street had an 80 percent survival rate, would that have an impact on which oncology group you personally chose for your care? It might. That powerful set of data also might cause the oncology group with an 80 percent score to figure out how to get to 90 percent. Or better.

We know right now that there is up to a 60 percent difference in the five-year mortality rates for breast cancer patients, depending on which hospital's surgical team did their actual surgery.[36] Those differences exist in the real world. If you are scheduled for surgery, would you like to know which surgeon had which survival rate? I suspect you would.

Those kinds of measures are possible, but only if we make a few key changes both in how we purchase and keep track of care. We need systems thinking and systems data in care delivery. A good place to start is with the four hard truths this chapter has introduced.

Let me remind you of those four hard truths we need to consider if we truly want to reform American health care. We need to keep in mind that 1 percent of our population uses 35 percent of our care dollars. We need to be very aware of the fact that care linkage deficiencies currently cripple our ability to deliver optimal care to far too many of our patients. Financial incentives in health care now too often work directly against optimal care. And we need to be aware that almost no one in health care thinks consistently, systematically, or even knows how to think systematically about major elements of real operational care improvement. There are notable and very encouraging exceptions, as you will read later, but that's the reality today for almost our entire American health care infrastructure.

With those four key facts of life as a foundation for our thinking, let's look at some tools we could use to improve care delivery in this country.

2

Data: The Missing Link for Health Care Reform

Over the past decade, major portions of the American economy have embraced a strong commitment to constant, effective, and consistent quality improvement. People in every major industry now clearly understand their industry's production processes in great detail, and people in key positions work constantly to use continuous process improvement techniques to reduce errors, cut costs, enhance product design, and improve functionality. Health care stands alone as the only major process-dependent industry where systematic process improvement is not embedded in the mind-sets of a wide range of major players, from frontline workers to operational managers to industry leaders.

As I noted in the last chapter, perverse market incentives and dysfunctional economic realities for American care providers create part of that problem. Health care is not incented in any effective way to measure the quality of care at multiple levels of performance and then use that information to continuously improve quality. The economic incentives for health care encourage and reward volumes of care, not improved outcomes of care. Those incentives need to be redesigned if we are going to optimize the delivery of care in America. Process reengineering will not happen on any scale in health care until there is a financial reward for doing exactly that. No industry reengineers just for the sheer pleasure of reengineering. It's too much work to do without a business model that makes reengineering a business imperative. Health care does not currently have that business model. In health care, as I noted earlier, successful process reengineering can actually do financial damage to a caregiver.

The frequently perverse economic incentives embedded in the current fee-for-service payment approach are not, however, the only major problem we face in making health care more effective and efficient in America. We actually have a bigger problem. Even if we all had the right financial incentive, most caregivers would not be able to achieve any real process reengineering success in American health care today because a major tool needed for reengineering simply does not exist in health care.

What is that tool?

Data. Health care lacks data.

How Other Industries Create Quality

Without data, care can't be engineered and caregivers can't be held truly accountable. Other industries who do reengineering as a routine fact of life all have data.

Look at GE. General Electric has absolutely world-class reengineering capabilities. GE is so good at designing and redesigning production facilities and processes that it actually sets a Six Sigma quality standard for itself. Six Sigma™ is a data-driven methodology designed to measure the error rate of any process. Table 2.1 shows the error rates that correspond to sigma levels. The goal of the method is to achieve no more than 3.4 errors per million opportunities. At GE, production processes typically make fewer than three errors per million units.

Three errors per million are not very many.

In health care, when some levels of quantifiable quality measures are actually available through reporting processes like HEDIS,[1] the gold standard for compliance—the rate that would get a plan a number one ranking—might be 88.6 percent. That is in fact the

Table 2.1. Sigma Levels and Error Rates.

Sigma Level	Defects per Million Opportunities	Error-Free Performance (%)
Six	3.4	99.9997
Five	230	99.98
Four	6,210	99.4
Three	66,800	93.3
Two	308,000	69.2
One	690,000	30.9

Source: A. Spanyi and M. Wurtzel. "Six Sigma for the Rest of Us." *Quality Digest*, July 2003. http://www.qualitydigest.com.

best score among all health plans in the country for breast cancer screening. Compliance with best practice at the 88.6 percent level means, of course, 11.4 percent noncompliance. This might seem like a small number until you do the math. The Six Sigma experts at GE, Motorola, 3M, McKesson, and many other corporations[2] would quickly point out that an 11.4 percent noncompliance level means 114,000 errors per million patients.

Compare 114,000 errors with three errors. That's a fairly major difference—and remember, 114,000 errors is the absolute best practice for the entire nation for that measurement. It's not the average score for all providers or even the minimally acceptable level of performance for all caregivers. It's the best. Look at the HEDIS performance chart in Table 2.2. Check out the top of the range performance levels and the average performance levels in each HEDIS measurement category. Average is not at all impressive. If an average performance for a particular HEDIS measure is 66.8 percent compliance (as it is for controlling hypertension), that represents 332,000 cases of noncompliance per million patients.

On a Six Sigma scale, that level is two sigma, as you can see in Table 2.3. Health care doesn't begin to approach Six Sigma levels for any of the major categories of quality and process measurement that currently exist.

Table 2.2 How Health Care Plans Vary in Performance by Selected HEDIS Measures.

HEDIS Measure[1]	10th Percentile Performance[2] (%)	Average Performance[3] (%)	90th Percentile Performance[4] (%)
Cholesterol management in heart attack patients	39.1	50.9	61.3
Screening for colorectal cancer	36.7	49.0	61.8
Screening for kidney disease in patients with diabetes	40.1	52.0	65.5
Controlling high blood pressure	56.2	66.8	75.4
Recommended treatment of acute depression	54.4	61.6	70.8
Screening for breast cancer	65.5	72.3	80.2

[1] HEDIS measures how often health plans offer care that complies with best practice guidelines.

[2] 10th percentile performance is the performance level at which a health plan outperforms 10 percent of all plans. A 10th percentile performance of 39.1 percent means that 10 percent of health plans managed cholesterol in 39.1 percent or less of heart attack patients.

[3] The average performance level for all health plans. On average, health plans managed cholesterol in 50.9 percent of heart attack patients.

[4] 90th percentile performance is the performance level at which a health plan outperforms 90 percent of all plans. A 90th percentile performance of 61.3 percent means that 90 percent of health plans managed cholesterol in 61.3 percent or less of heart attack patients.

Sources: National Committee for Quality Assurance. "The State of Health Care Quality 2005: Industry Trends and Analysis." Washington D.C.: National Committee for Quality Assurance, 2006, Table 9; National Committee for Quality Assurance. "Quality Compass 2006." Washington D.C.: National Committee for Quality Assurance, 2006.

Table 2.3. How Health Care Plan Performance Looks in a Six Sigma World.

HEDIS Measure	10th Percentile Performance	Average Performance	90th Percentile Performance
Cholesterol management in heart attack patients	1.2 sigma	1.6 sigma	1.8 sigma
Screening for colorectal cancer	1.2	1.5	1.9
Screening for kidney disease in patients with diabetes	1.3	1.6	1.9
Controlling high blood pressure	1.7	2.0	2.2
Recommended treatment of acute depression	1.7	1.8	2.1
Screening for breast cancer	1.9	2.1	2.4

Note: HEDIS measures how often health plans offer care that complies with best practice guidelines.

So how does GE actually get to those excellent Six Sigma results? It's not by simply working extremely hard. It's not just by having well-trained, highly motivated people, each individually trying to do the right thing. If that approach were enough, health care would be at Six Sigma right now. Health care has a lot of very well-trained, completely well-intentioned, fully committed, extremely hard-working people—who now make up to 114,000 errors per million patients in some of the very best and highest quality care settings.

So good intentions are not enough . . . at GE or in health care. How does GE actually get the job done? With a quality improvement process called MAIC.[3] That basic MAIC process is done at GE over and over again. Every production employee at GE knows that process. Highly trained individuals, who have the title of Six

Sigma Black Belts, guarantee that the process will be consistently followed at GE.

What do those four letters "MAIC" stand for?

1. Measurement
2. Analysis
3. Improvement
4. Control

Each of the four MAIC steps is essential to the success of the effort. Without any one of them, the Six Sigma effort at GE would fail. Each step must be done in turn. That's important to remember. First things first—each step in its turn.

So what is the first step?

Data. The essence of Step 1 is data. Clear, available, accurate, current, and complete data about the process being reengineered is essential. Without that data, the entire GE Six Sigma process would fail. GE cannot start at Step 2. Measurement must precede analysis. Data is first.

As I noted in Chapter One, health care has a truly amazing data deficit. That's a real problem. It's impossible to measure care outcomes, care consequences, or basic care processes without data. The simple act of measuring, by definition, requires some form of data. This really is a key point to understand. Health care's lack of data is the fundamental flaw that undermines and cripples the whole concept of using Six Sigma or other equivalent continuous quality improvement (CQI) theories and practices to significantly improve health care. Health care doesn't have the necessary data to do that work.

Paper Records Don't Deliver Good Data

Why does health care lack data? Again, this is a logical and basic point of fact that we all need to understand if we truly want to reform health care in America. Health care lacks data because the primary source of data for health care in America today is still the paper medical record. According to a recent study funded by the Robert Wood Johnson Foundation, fewer than one in ten doctors makes use of electronic medical records. As few as 5 percent of hospitals use computerized physician order entry, the simplest form of electronic record keeping.[4]

Health data in America is made up of separate pieces of paper. Many separate pieces of paper. A paper medical record is kept in a file drawer by each caregiver for each patient. If a patient with comorbidities has three doctors, there are typically three separate paper medical records—each kept in a separate filing system, generally in three different and unconnected buildings.

Here are some basic facts about paper records:

- *Paper medical records tend to be incomplete.* If a patient changes doctors, those records are even more incomplete. The records are split between the doctors.
- *Paper medical records are not uniform.* They come in many shapes, sizes, and formats. Everyone who provides care can invent his or her own. The pieces of paper that result often don't compare well with each other. Even the data definitions have too often tended to be site-specific for many data elements. Some of the paper records are literally illegible—handwritten by physicians.
- *Paper medical records are isolated.* The pieces of paper sit physically in each provider office. Isolated. Isolated from each other and even from the caregivers who treat the patients. The separate and individual paper files generated by each provider are generally not available to other care providers—certainly not in any consistent way.
- *Paper medical records are inert.* In an era of interactive databases, paper records are completely passive. Obviously, paper files cannot and do not interact with the doctor in any active way to point out, for example, potentially troublesome test result trends that probably need to be studied. The paper files also don't point out that the drug just prescribed by a given physician shouldn't be

given to a particular patient who had previously been prescribed another drug by another physician.

In a science-based profession where decisions and treatment plans are supposed to be based on full information and current science, the actual paper-based information storage approach is antiquated and horribly flawed. In this nonsystem, care providers' ability to do good ongoing science and research about what really works is obviously badly impaired.

Other than trying to use pure, unassisted human memory, without even pieces of paper to serve as a partial reminder, it's hard to imagine a more dysfunctional way of storing, holding, and using detailed and valuable medical information.

As a data storage strategy, the paper medical record is massively flawed. Remember how care linkage deficiencies happen in American health care. A patient with two diseases will often have two doctors. Since two doctors writing two prescriptions generally do not interact and also have two separate paper files for their care site medical records, the first prescription that was written for the patient is too often totally unknown to the second doctor who writes the second prescription. Adverse drug events (ADEs) are the most common cause of medical errors in hospitalized patients. Roughly 5 percent of patients experience a medication error.[5] Although not all medication errors cause harm, many do—and in addition to the human costs, they can add 20 percent to the cost of the hospital stay.[6] Doctors who use paper medical records have no way of preventing ADEs unless the patient can recall his own prescription history. Each year, more than 700,000 people are treated for adverse drug events in emergency rooms in the United States; unintentional overdoses are the most common problem.[7] Perhaps not all of those events could be eliminated by better data availability—but most very definitely could.

It's a pretty sad state of data availability and use.

The paper files are inert, incomplete, and very often literally inaccessible. They definitely do not let our caregivers give us the best care possible.

We Need Electronic Data to Measure Performance

Paper records make it nearly impossible to evaluate caregiver performance. When the RAND researchers did their wonderful work to figure out how well the American care infrastructure is doing to meet the needs of patients, a team of twenty nurses worked to examine and recode every single separate medical file from every single care provider for those seven thousand patients.[8] It was Herculean work that created a badly needed statistical insight into the state of American health care delivery.

We now have some valid, quantifiable performance data because of that RAND study. That's the good news. The bad news is that the extremely important database from the RAND study is entirely static—a snapshot, frozen in time. Three years later, we have no way of knowing whether any of those alarming care patterns have gotten better or worse. We'd need to assign another team of nurses to go out into the field to pull the current set of paper files for those seven thousand patients to give us another snapshot report. And then, even if we had all of those nurses do all of that manual work all over again, we'd actually have only two data points rather than one. Two is quite a bit better than one, but are two data points really enough to track how America is spending $2 trillion on care?

This lack of data makes real process reengineering in health care impossible. Process reengineering requires a process to reengineer. It requires clear data about the outcome of each process and clear data about the inputs to each process. We can't fix the error rate in the production of hubcaps without a clear measurement of the initial error rate in producing hubcaps. We can't measure the impact of any changes in the hubcap production process without carefully measuring and understanding each step of the current production process. Reengineering is a science. Medical processes now are an art—unmeasured at the results end and undocumented and unmeasured in their preresult process components and steps.

So improving outcomes by improving process in health care tends not to happen; and when it does, the learning is not shared. At one American hospital, a rare continuous improvement process took the number of steps needed to fill a prescription from 17 to 5, cut the time to process the prescription from 92 minutes to 17 minutes, and cut the number of potentially dangerous errors made in the process by 90 percent.[9] Patient lives were protected. Costs were eliminated. Process improved. But that entire process improvement approach has remained limited to that setting—with no process in place to spread the same learning to other sites of care.

We need data to chart outcomes in order to improve the process that creates those outcomes.

Patients need that data to exist. At the physician level, where care decisions are made and patients choose their care providers, because of the paper medical record we don't have the data necessary to track which providers or care teams have achieved the best results for back surgery, knee surgery, or eye surgery. We don't know which oncology group gives patients the longest survival time from Stage II lung cancer, or who does the best job of treating breast cancer and getting it into remission. None of that comparative data is available now. Oncology groups don't know how their success rates compare to other oncology groups. How can the providers with the worst performance levels improve when they have no sense at all that their below-average performance levels could and should be improved?

That total void of performance-based quantifiable information is a data tragedy. It definitely explains why Six Sigma performance improvement doesn't exist in health care. We don't have the fundamental base-level data necessary to do that work.

And we need that data so we can get about the business of systematically improving care.

We Need Electronic Data for Better Care

So what could be done to get that data? The good news is that a tool exists that could give us full, accurate, quick, and extremely useful access to that data. At the risk of sounding flip, that tool is called a computer. The jury is in on that point. We need computers. Paper files and paper medical records will never do the job. They functionally and logistically simply cannot ever do that job. Sorting and resorting multiple paper files simply can never give us the data we need to reengineer care. Or even to track care performance. Computerized data is needed to track health care performance, improve health care process, and keep doctors informed about patient care; it can be used to improve health care in literally thousands of ways.

So if we do want systematic care improvement in this country, we obviously need to computerize America's medical records. It's really just common sense, particularly when we use computers so fully in every other business and profession. If we had a computerized database for health care, we wouldn't need to wait another decade for RAND to do a second laborious and totally manual chart review to see how well or badly the American health care nonsystem is currently performing.

With a fully computerized database, we could aggregate data electronically and duplicate the national RAND study in every community every week—and we could track progress on key care performance levels in community after community at a level that would lend itself to real process improvement. We could give doctors interactive electronic tools to help remind each physician of potential dangerous drug interactions at the critically important point in time when prescriptions are written. Computer programs could also advise the doctor about lab test findings and their potential significance, and even remind physicians of the best current science for a particular condition. The computer could also very easily and consistently trigger specific reminders for doctors about what care steps are needed next for a particular condition for a particular patient. If we want to create better, more consistent care, that information needs to be easily available to doctors in ways that can be achieved only by a computer.

Lawyers, architects, and engineers all use computerized information regularly in their daily work. Their work has gotten better as a result. It's time for doctors to have that same set of profession-enhancing tools.

So how can we get these tools to doctors? At the risk of sounding simplistic, the very best way to computerize health care information is to completely replace the paper medical record with a computerized medical record in each hospital and physician office. This is now possible. Multiple computer systems now exist that can accomplish that task. The hardest lifting on initial automated medical record system thinking, design, functionality, and availability is now behind us. Quite a few vendors sell very workable electronic medical record systems. A few sell excellent systems. That first formidable logistical hurdle has now been cleared. Those systems will each get better over time, but they are good enough now. The goal now needs to be to get those systems in place as quickly as possible in as many provider sites as possible.

We've definitely made that particular commitment at Kaiser Permanente. We've made that commitment for the reasons described above. We are investing heavily in complete electronic medical records for all of our care—clinical, hospital, and even in-home nursing care. That electronic data will help us improve care and it will give us an incredible research window into the efficiency and efficacy of care. We are putting those systems in place as I write this book.

Many other American care providers are going down similar paths. Large multispecialty medical groups such as the Mayo Clinic, Cleveland Clinic, Intermountain Healthcare, and Geisinger Health

Systems have all made the commitment to put electronic medical records (EMRs) in place. Many major hospital systems are moving toward electronic records, and many smaller clinics and solo practice physicians are also on that path. But the smaller care sites are moving toward EMRs at a much slower pace—a pace so slow that we will not get to a fully automated American care infrastructure for more than a decade.[10] That pace may increase substantially if we providers are required to submit claims electronically and if new vendors figure out how to support new EMRs for the solo practice doctors. But that has not yet happened, so experts continue to predict a decade before everyone in health care is "wired."

I'll return to that point later. It's important to understand those time frames. A decade is too long for the health care reform that this country needs.

It's also important to recognize that simply automating the old paper record is a very good first step, but it's really only a very first step. Scanning documents or directly inputting data into an electronic database creates a computerized record, but it does not create a record that can meet Six Sigma goals. It doesn't automatically create electronic linkages between multiple providers. The mere act of automating data in a medical office is not a silver bullet that automatically improves care.

Electronic Records Are a Caregiver Support Tool

Ideally, to maximize the positive impact on care, the electronic medical record tool should be more than a simple record-keeping device for the physician. It should be an interactive tool that helps the physician improve care. Our motto at Kaiser Permanente on that point is "Make the right thing easy to do."

Computers should be a direct physician practice support tool. Computer programs can and should remind doctors of needed care for individual patients. Computers can also help each doctor communicate electronically with individual patients. The opportunities are immense. Computer-supported care will be better care. Computers today have immense potential to add value to care delivery in multiple ways.

As noted earlier, systematically detecting potential adverse drug-to-drug interactions for individual patients is a relatively simple process for a computer to handle. In one medical process reengineering pilot at Kaiser Permanente designed to prevent adverse drug events, we went beyond simple drug-to-drug interaction.

We used a computerized system to monitor people receiving a common and potent type of drug, anticoagulants. The margin between an effective anticoagulant dose and a dangerous dose is very small. We created a computerized system to monitor lab values to make sure that our patients were receiving the right doses and to stop those drugs before surgery.

How big were the dividends? Big. The risk of death from complications or failures of these medications decreased by 77 percent.[11]

The basic approach used by the doctors in this study was pure process improvement in the Six Sigma tradition. Baseline data about anticoagulation complication rates was created. For a given patient population on anticoagulants, the number of historical bleeding complications was measured. That measurement of bleeding complications created a performance floor. Then the management process was reengineered, using the computer as a tool. Prior measurements and analysis had shown that a significant portion of patients experienced bleeding or clotting problems from either too much or too little of the anticoagulant drugs. That was a key piece of data.

So what was done with that information? The reengineering process that followed was pretty simple: the computers were programmed by a team of pharmacologists to monitor patients on anticoagulants. A team of pharmacy professionals with specialized knowledge in anticoagulant therapy was formed to follow these patients by phone. Patients and pharmacists worked together, with the support and blessing of physicians, to make sure that necessary lab tests were performed and followed and that doses were adjusted as needed. When patients were scheduled for surgery, they were proactively and strategically taken off the dangerous prescription.

How well did that level of care-process reengineering work?

As I noted earlier, nearly 80 percent of fatal complications or failures of these potent medications went away. The results were exceptional. And quick. It was a great learning experience.

That whole approach doesn't feel to the average patient like one-of-a-kind rocket science. It feels like a pretty basic and logical operational concept with a high reward factor. You'd expect everyone in health care to do that same process. They would if they could. But most cannot—particularly if they are limited entirely to paper medical records.

In surgical settings without that computerized tool in place, most surgeons too often simply do not even know exactly what prescriptions their patients are actually taking. Why is that? Because surgeons perform surgery. Think about how health care is typically "organized." Surgeons do not prescribe. Internists prescribe. Surgeons cut. Surgeons aren't internists. Or pediatricians. That's just how things work in health care. Remember the issue of care linkage deficiencies. The surgeons almost always are not the doctors who initially prescribed the various medications taken by each patient, since surgeons are not, by role, function, or training, "prescribing" doctors. That's fine. We really don't want all of our prescriptions written by surgeons. But we do want surgeons to know all of the prescriptions that have been written for their patients.

Since surgeons in this country also far too often do not get to see all of their patients' actual presurgery primary care paper medical records—records that are created by—and stored by—the patients' primary care doctors—most surgeons have to rely on their patients to somehow remember and then share their own prescription information. The normal and generally accepted presurgical preparation approach in this country is literally to expect each patient—often a seriously ill patient—to tell all of that information to the surgeon. That is a highly imperfect process, at best.

Even in those cases where the surgeon does know about all of a given patient's medications, the surgeons may not be aware that an unintended consequence for a particular medication could be bleeding challenges during surgery. Surgeons are not pharmacists. Practically speaking, they do not and cannot know every potential effect or impact of every available drug. But a computer can be programmed to know that those potential complicating consequences exist, and a computer can be programmed to warn the surgeon.

In this test case, as I noted earlier, the patients all were served by a multispecialty medical group that used a common computerized medical record for all patients. So the surgeons in the group could simply have the computer check the full medical record to see what medications the patients were on. If those particular patients had not been in that computer supported care setting, 79 percent more patients would have had bleeding complications during surgery.

The advantage to patients of systems thinking and full data availability on the part of all relevant caregivers was pretty obvious in this study. Without that kind of interactive computerized data, the number of surgical deaths will stay up and the rate of surgical complications will increase, rather than get better. That lack of information flow on behalf of the patient creates some of the typical care linkage deficiencies that happen all over America every day in the surgery area. Only an interactive, computerized process can add a whole array of presurgery safety features consistent with the best surgical care.

Shouldn't every patient going into major surgery have that level of protection? Of course.

Five to ten years from now, people will look back on the paucity of information sharing that results in today's world from America's overwhelming reliance on a paper medical record and will consider this to be medical dark ages. New medical students as early as five years from now will not believe that anyone could ever have practiced medicine with so little access to necessary information.

Remember, the reduction in bleeding complications happened in this study because the caregivers used available data in a Six Sigma–type of process improvement project to reengineer a piece of care delivery to solve a measurable problem. In the process, they used a computer to assist the caregiver in ways that can't be easily or consistently done without the computer. They also used data to measure adverse results and to tie those adverse results to particular causality. Process thinking tied to scientific thinking is an incredibly powerful combination. We need to use that combination in health care a lot more often.

Electronic Records Are Critical for Process Thinking

Any continuous quality improvement (CQI) or Six Sigma expert would find the learnings from that project to be extremely basic. Even simple. But, as I noted earlier, that kind of CQI thinking is new to health care.

I know that I am repeating myself a bit here, but this is important information relative to how care is delivered. A health care delivery system that does not measure and evaluate its own performance is doomed to make, at best, only marginal improvements in that performance. When performance is measured, significant improvement can result. In one of the Kaiser Permanente pilot studies we did in part to evaluate the various ways computers could be used to support better care, we put together a computerized checklist of activities that needed to be done for patients with kidney failure. By putting together a multidisciplinary team and reminding the caregivers of what care each kidney patient needed on each visit, patients experienced fewer hospital days than did the population of comparable kidney patients outside the Kaiser Permanente system. The death rate among patients in the program was half that of kidney failure patients in the larger community.[12] That approach used a basic process improvement tool kit to look at what patient and provider reminders were needed and then created a computer-supported process to get those reminders to each of the caregivers at the point of care. Lives were saved.

Computer-supported care worked.

The list of possible improvement areas is almost infinite. Look at detecting breast cancer as another example of the systematic use of data to support care improvement. The most common quality measurement today in breast cancer detection is whether or not a woman has recently received a mammogram. That is, in fact, a very useful process measure relative to breast cancer detection. The national HEDIS quality standards we discussed earlier have been used to look at health plan mammography rates. American women are much better off because the success rate of health plans in getting high percentages of women to have mammograms is both measured and publicly reported through HEDIS. That is one of the areas where existing externally imposed measurement requirements have helped care levels improve measurably. But now we need to go to the next level. We need to know how well the mammograms were done.

That simple HEDIS measurement of how many women actually received a mammogram basically assumes that all mammograms are done at essentially the same level of quality. Most people assume that all mammograms are equal. That assumption was made with no specific data. In fact, studies have demonstrated distinct differences between radiologists' ability to identify cancer, particularly in the early stage, on mammograms. Mammograms are really hard to read; in many cases, skill levels vary. In one study, a panel of radiologists interpreted mammograms from women who were already known to either have cancer or be cancer-free; different radiologists interpreted mammograms differently more than 20 percent of the time.[13] The study had two phases, and the radiologists read the same films on two separate occasions.

Variability in reading mammograms results both in further testing for women who don't have cancer—and in missed cancers. Ten percent of radiologists in the study recommended further testing in only 75 percent of the women who actually had cancer. That means your cancer would have been missed one quarter of the time, if your mammogram had been read by a radiologist at that screening level.

Again, anyone versed in CQI or Six Sigma would know what to do next—gather more data to get a really good sense of whether or not a performance problem existed and, if it did, use the data to figure out the exact nature of the problem. That kind of analysis was done. It proved to be very useful.

In that pilot program, the senior radiologist, aware that some cancers were being missed by radiologists, looked at their records, counted the cancers they missed, and printed their averages on charts and graphs. Those missing too many cancers were either let go or reassigned. Those radiologists who didn't read enough mammograms to keep their skill levels high were required to read more. Today, the pilot radiology team has a mandatory three-times-a-year test to hone their interpretation skills—and they miss many fewer cancers. Now, on a broader level, within the system, the work of mammogram interpretation is limited to those with the ability to read well.[14]

That approach saved lives. It's also simply good, quality-based systems improvement thinking applied to health care. That is not, however, how most of health care works. Certainly not for mammograms. If you personally get a mammogram right now, today, you have no way of knowing if the person reading your mammogram is at the highest detection level—or is likely to let 50 percent more cases slip by to Stage III status. Since Stage III cancer has a five-year survival rate that is 20 percent lower than early-stage cancers, that 50 percent detection difference could be very directly relevant to your life.[15]

We shouldn't need to debate this point. Health care needs many levels of performance data. We all need it to improve care and make decisions about care. I met relatively recently with a national conference of hospital leaders. The audience contained senior hospital executives from some of the best hospitals in America. I pointed out to them that if any of the hospital leaders in the room was diagnosed that afternoon with a potentially terminal cancer, they would not even know which of the oncologists in their own hospital have a 60 percent cure rate for that particular cancer and which oncologists have only a 30 percent cure rate. Even as nationally known hospital leaders—senior hands-on health care executives—they do not and would not know that key piece of information in a way that could directly affect their own personal survival. We do know that significant performance differences exist. Every study of care outcomes shows real differences and significant variations in actual performance levels and success. But we don't track those performance differences systematically and then use those differences to figure out how to systematically improve care.

We need data in American health care so that performance can be measured. We need data so that care can be reengineered. We need data so that we can set Six Sigma standards for ourselves in key areas of care and then attain them.

You can argue—and should argue—that one reason for the fact that data do not exist already is that caregivers have no economic incentive that either require or reward that use of data. So the relevant data is not collected. It's a chicken-and-egg argument at one level. Which comes first? Data? Or incentives that drive the creation of data? When sufficient incentives or disincentives exist, data can and will be generated.

Anyone who truly wants to reengineer and improve care should have the insight to know that the availability of data is foundational to care improvement and should therefore put market-based strategies in place that both reward and require the existence of that data. As you will read later, I believe the buyers will need to insist on that approach or it will not happen. We've already proven that it will not happen if left to the sole control of the care community. I also believe that when the data is available, the scope of uses for that data will explode—and uses will exist that aren't even dreamed of today. But today, we have perverse financial incentives, paper medical records, and no data.

Without data, Six Sigma thinking is impossible. We all need to recognize the key fact that probably the single most important reason why CQI processes have not been used in health care is the almost total lack of usable data about relative health care processes. We need to fix that data void as quickly as we can. I'll suggest alternative ways we might do that fairly quickly in a couple of pages. Before we get to that point, we first need to understand the potential for real Six Sigma thinking in health care.

Six Sigma Can Be a Legitimate Care Goal

Some people contend that applying any standards even remotely resembling Six Sigma to health care providers is a stupid and unworkable idea because health care is a much more complex and inherently much messier process than the production of a television set or the building of a car. Critics also argue that people building a car do not have to rely on the car to voluntarily take a prescription, accept an implant, or lose weight.

"We can't achieve Six Sigma results," a lot of caregivers will say, "because we must deal with individual patients, and patients are impossible to control. We can't force our patients to take their medication, for example, so we can't be held accountable as caregivers for the results of medication-dependent care at Six Sigma performance levels."

Those are true observations. Health care involves patients as well as caregivers, and patients have their own free will, so Six Sigma goals for some issues and some objectives are in fact impossible to achieve. We can't ever force all patients to do anything. Nor should we. So Six Sigma applied directly to patient behavior is a bad idea.

Those anti–Six Sigma folks are not, however, entirely accurate in saying that health care therefore should be held to a much lower standard of performance. There actually are a number of ways of creating valid and useful Six Sigma performance levels in health care without having to expect patients to adhere to Six Sigma standards. It's not, as many caregivers say, totally impossible. The challenge is to figure out exactly what type of performance can and should be held to that standard.

So what Six Sigma measure could we use? What should health care be accountable for doing with absolute consistency? Here is the simple guideline: health care should be accountable for what the caregivers do.

Provider compliance, not patient compliance, should be the Six Sigma goal.

We need to be accountable for specific elements of doctor and care team performance, not for absolute patient compliance. Appropriate standards of pure physician and care system performance can be defined. How can that be done? A perfectly workable standard approach is to set up specific processes that create absolutely consistent provider team activities relative to the care offered to each patient with a given condition.

Let's go back to the breast cancer example. Holding caregivers accountable by Six Sigma standards for whether every woman in a patient population actually received a mammogram is unfair and impossible. Mammograms in our society are voluntary. Voluntary means that people can say no. And some always will. Another measurement is needed. Instead of patient compliance, we need to measure relevant caregiver performance. Measuring whether every single woman in the population was actually offered a mammogram by the care system is, by contrast, a controllable and measurable activity. A given care team could very legitimately be held to Six Sigma standards relative to whether every single woman on their relevant patient list was actually given the opportunity and choice of having a mammogram at least once every two years.

Getting every person who has diabetes to actually undergo an eye exam is an unfair and unreasonable Six Sigma standard. But offering every single person with diabetes in a given population an eye exam is a fully workable standard and the "offering rate" should be subject to Six Sigma measurements and expectations. We can and should measure how many patients actively received eye exams, and we should set up reward systems relative to that measure, but patient compliance will never reach Six Sigma levels. Provider performance can, however, reach those levels.

If we hold the care system accountable for specific activities that are clearly under the control of the care system, we can say that our Six Sigma goal for every single patient going into surgery is to have our computer check all prior prescriptions to see if any drugs currently prescribed for the patient might cause severe bleeding. The care system can't always prevent the bleeding, but an interactive computer program can potentially check whether a patient might have been prescribed a known dangerous drug, and it can send an alert to the patient's surgeon. Every patient. All prescriptions. Scout for any with known potential bleeding implications. Those are all measures that lead themselves to Six Sigma accountability goals. Many lives would be saved in America if that particular standard was met.

Six Sigma can be done in health care. We just need to be very clear about what we measure. Measurement is foundational to that process.

That brings us back to data.

The key to introducing Six Sigma and process improvement approaches to health care will be to generate the data needed to measure performance through a computerized system.

We definitely need electronically available data as soon as possible so that health care buyers can finally act like buyers act in other industries: making value-based purchases and rewarding the best caregivers and the best care systems with purchases and volume.

Electronic Medical Records Are the Gold Standard

So how can that be done? It is, I believe, possible if we aim carefully for exactly the right use of available data. As I noted earlier, the very best way of getting health care performance data in a comprehensive form is the automated electronic medical record. As I've described, the technology for creating an electronic medical record already exists. It works. It can be done—and should be done—everywhere. In a multispecialty medical group setting, a single electronic medical record can contain all of the clinical information about each patient, including the actual scores from every lab test. Ideally, this electronic record can hold the full digital images from every X-ray and scan. That's the gold standard for medical information. But not all caregivers will be able to move quickly enough to achieve that standard.

EMRs require significant investments. The solo practitioners and small medical groups that make up the majority of health care providers in this country can agree that EMRs improve safety, but they don't see an immediate financial benefit to investing in them. They don't have a dollar incentive to change.[16]

EMRs also require a nonmonetary investment. They represent a whole new way of recording care information for each caregiver. The caregivers involved generally need to go through a change of practice experience that has all of the temporary stress points that any significant change of process creates. Transitions are always hard. They are particularly challenging for professionals in any setting who are used to doing their jobs in a particular way. We need those transitions to a computerized database to happen, however, and so that process needs to happen wherever and whenever it can.

Once through the process, the caregivers tend to love the new power and information flow that results from electronic records, so the pain of transition is replaced by pure professional gratification fairly quickly once the system is fully in place.

In a very few years, I believe doctors will look back on today's information deficits and wonder how anyone practiced medicine without electronic medical records and computerized support. New physicians will say to old physicians, "Did you really have to figure out two thousand potential drug interactions in your head? Did you really not know what the lab results were if another doctor ran the tests? Wow, that must have been frustrating—even scary." The old doctors will ask themselves the same questions. These electronic tools are needed—and they are needed now. That investment needs to be made. But that won't happen everywhere overnight. So what do we do for the meantime? That's the next chapter.

3

What Do We Do Until the Electronic Medical Record Arrives?

Computerizing the database for American health care is obviously the right strategy for health care reform. However, we need to be honest with ourselves as both policy strategists and operational logisticians about the reality that the electronic medical record will not happen overnight for all American caregivers. It's a badly needed tool, but it is a tool that will take a while to get in place everywhere.

Changing all caregivers from a paper system to an electronic system will take both money and time—as much as fifteen years and $115 billion.[1] The large multispecialty medical practices are already moving very quickly in that direction, but most caregivers in independent and solo practices are moving much more slowly. New versions of EMRs specially designed to accommodate solo practice doctors will inevitably emerge in a world of constantly evolving and highly competitive systems development and marketing, but these systems are not available right now. Most caregivers will not be on electronic systems for quite a few years. That's a scary thing. We really can't afford to wait that long to initiate real health care reform—so the question we need to ask ourselves is this: Is there a quicker way to get a big part of that job done? Can we move more quickly to create access to computerized information about care?

Accelerating the pace of EMR rollout is logistically and economically challenging if not impossible, so if we decide we want computerized data now to improve patient care, we obviously need an interim step. Does that step exist?

Electronic Claims-Based Medical Data Can Help

The answer is yes. The good news is that a fully electronic medical record with a complete history of all care delivered to each individual patient is not the only possible interactive electronic data source we can create and utilize for improving health care. The EMR is obviously the best and most complete source. The paper medical record is equally obviously the worst source. In between paper and the EMR, there actually is another potentially very valuable partial database that can be made available to us in a computerized format relatively soon.

I believe we need to take advantage of that opportunity. That new electronic database can, I believe, do enough real work relative to both care performance measurement and caregiver information linkages that we will be able to get the next generation of health care reform on the road. It's obvious that we need electronic data. It's equally obvious that we can't get it soon enough in a complete medical record format from all caregivers. So we need to get access to the second best set of care-related computerized data, and we need to use that data to begin the process of improving care. There is some irony in the fact that electronic data about the vast majority of American patients actually exists now—but it's not in the computers of doctors or hospitals.

So who exactly has that data on their computers? Payers. The really interesting news is that a very sizable electronic database about care sits today on the computers of the various payers—the organizations who now pay the actual claims that create the primary revenue source for American health care today. Specific payers who now have extensive electronic data on their computers include health plans, health insurers, and the various government programs that pay claims to providers on behalf of the patients they insure.

Box 3.1. Evolution of Automated Record Availability.

Jay Crosson, M.D., executive director,
Permanente Federation

The book assumes that the personal health record (PHR) database will be needed for short-term health care reform because the more comprehensive automated medical record system will not be available quickly enough for most American providers. It's not hard to envision an alternative time frame where the new PHR agenda combined with the requirement from all private and public payers that providers submit their claims electronically will inspire systems vendors to step forward very quickly with new, less expensive, externally hosted shared electronic medical record (EMR) system products. Since the providers soon will need to send claims electronically to payers, it's not a huge step for the electronic billing system vendors to become mini-EMR vendors. The mini-EMR vendors could interact with each other and also could be designed to tap into the new PHR database for some of their data. If that happens, the pace of the EMR rollout could be accelerated hugely—to the point where most solo physicians end up with EMRs very quickly. It will be a new world.

Those payment files are already on computers and they already contain both financial data and quite a bit of medical data.

Why do insurers have medical information on their computers? Simply to pay claims. Insurers and other payers will not pay a claim today unless the claim form sent by the provider to the insurer lists the exact provider who did the service, the specific care procedure that was done for the patient, and the specific diagnosis for the patient that justified the care. Providers of care send that level of relatively detailed medical data every single day to insurers to get money. The payers put that medical data in their computers. That data is in those computers right now, waiting to be used. Right now, with very few exceptions, that data is not being used to support the delivery of care.

Siloed Claims Data

A number of factors have combined very nicely and very recently to turn that existing claims payment database of insurers into a database that could begin to assist in reforming and improving health care. Those new developments relative to American health care data input and accessibility are described here and in Chapter Four. The important thing to recognize now relative to health care reform is that there is a lot of data in those payer computers. Important data. We can now build a very useful electronic data service based on the computerized information about individual patients' diagnoses and procedures that is already being collected and stored by the existing payment systems for both the health insurance industry and by all of the government agencies that pay claims for Medicare, Medicaid, and related entitlement programs.

To be useful, the data will need to be aggregated a bit and brought together in a systematic way. Right now, that data sits on a thousand different computers—each payer with their own machines and their own computer files. The current splintered electronic data storage situation for insurance payers is more than a bit like the similarly siloed storage approach used by care providers for paper medical records—with each paper file sitting in a different file cabinet in a different office. The extremely important difference between those two "silo" problems is, however, that the paper medical record in the doctor's office is inherently and irrevocably isolated and inert, while the various payer databases are all electronic, computerized, and very capable of being both interactive and electronically aggregated. Computers can be taught to share information. Paper files cannot. It's a pretty important difference.

That existing electronic claims information database is, therefore, potentially very useful if we think of it strategically. There are some challenges that need to be dealt with, of course. That claims data is on a lot of computers. Anyone working with computers knows that simply being digitized is not sufficient to create automatic interoperability or even to allow for simple and useful data sharing and aggregation. Some work needs to be done to make sharing of data possible. One major reason that the electronic claims database has never been regarded as a potentially useful tool for either health care improvement or measuring care system accountability is that the various payer databases have historically been quite different from each other and therefore extremely difficult to aggregate. That is changing, as you read this.

Unique Provider Number

That data is now becoming far more valuable and useful than it used to be, because a new federal law has required the use of a single and unique provider number for every single licensed physician and caregiver in America.[2]

That new, simple single provider identification number requirement has massive positive implications. One is that data between payers can now be aggregated by provider to show total patterns of care by each provider. In the old days, with three dozen payers in any market, the database for each payer might have only one-thirtieth of the actual performance information for each caregiver. It's hard to get strategically relevant and statistically valid data about how a given provider takes care of asthma patients if a given payer only has one-thirtieth of that provider's asthma patients in their payment data file. But if the data can be aggregated across payers to track total provider performance for all patients, then it's possible to get statistically valid and credible indications of provider performance. The old payer databases with separate provider numbers used by each payer for each physician made each individual payer's data files about each individual caregiver almost useless for monitoring and assessing overall care. Aggregated data could be far more useful.

The requirement that every provider have a single and unique number is a hugely important data breakthrough. Every payer used to invent its own ID code for each provider. When the data about how a given physician did relative to treating individual patients was on a hundred different payer systems with a hundred "unique" ID numbers used for any single doctor, the data about any single doctor could not be used in any effective aggregated way to look at overall care patterns or performance. That data also couldn't be used to help patients create a longitudinal history of their own care. Patients tend to change insurers fairly often. Some insurers have an annual 20 percent churn rate in their membership—as people move, change jobs, or simply decide to buy different coverage.[3] In the old days, each move of their coverage instantly truncated the payer database for each insured person. Claims data could not and did not follow the patient, both because no one was interested in maintaining continuous data on each patient and because provider identification codes were so different from payer to payer. But with a single national identification number for each provider, that situation has changed entirely.

If a major goal of the total health care reform process is to quickly and significantly improve community, caregiver, and patient access to relevant current and historical data about both individual patients and individual providers, as well as providing useful data about aggregate community care performance and processes as quickly as possible, then we will need to begin the integration and aggregation of the payer databases as quickly as possible. When that is done and all payers are using the same ID numbers for each physician, then the total body of electronic care-based information available today on the computerized claims payment databases of the large payers can actually be of very real use very quickly.

An Untapped Treasure

It's an untapped treasure. Those databases represent a vast wealth of information that has been functionally unusable and unavailable for care improvement and health care market reform purposes until now. It's a whole new way of looking at that data. Up to now, that array of data has been collected by payers and then used almost exclusively to pay claims. It has also been used to some degree by insurance actuaries in each company to track their historic claims payment expense trends and to help estimate future insurance costs. To a small degree, some of that data has already helped guide some of the early care management processes for some health plans. A few independent care management companies also now are beginning to rely on the claims database of the payers and employers to detect opportunities to influence specific patients or their care.

But at this point, we have barely tapped the larger potential of that database. We have not created community-wide databases to tell us how well we are doing on diabetic care in New Orleans or New Brunswick. We haven't screened the total claims payment performance data for an entire community to see which kids have not yet been immunized—or which kids haven't recently refilled their asthma prescriptions. A more aggressive agenda for systematic and consistent use of that claims-based data ought to be a top policy priority both for health care reformers and for the companies that purchase health care coverage for their employees.

It's important to recognize what is already in that claims payment database. It has a relatively complete set of recent data on each patient, listing all providers used by the patient along with all diagnosis done for the patient. It has all current procedures, all current prescriptions, and a list of recent lab tests run for the patient. Because the actual computerized database is compiled by each payer, not by each individual care provider, it has full claims-level data for each patient relative to all providers who file claims for treating that patient. So the database is more complete than a solo provider paper medical record could ever be.

The claims-based record is not an electronic health record in the full sense of the term. It doesn't have actual lab test results. Some of the coding is flawed. The data is not current, up to the minute, like a good EMR. And, as I noted earlier, when people change health plans or insurers, that payer data has always been completely truncated for each patient by each carrier change. But the claims-based array of data is a lot better than nothing, and the issue of data truncation can and will be dealt with systematically in the near future by the payer community, by creating a process that will allow individual patients to switch their database electronically from payer to payer when the patients change health plans or health insurers. The payer industry has very recently agreed to make that data transferability service available to all patients. It's in the process of being implemented.

To make use of that data as quickly and completely as possible, we will need, as a society, to create a uniform data set about electronic personal health records. We need uniform data transfer requirements to be applied to all private and public payers in health care. If we really want to use that claims-based data most effectively, we need to end the truncation problem that happens when people change insurers by implementing easily usable data continuity strategies and approaches that all payers follow.

Electronic Health Records and Patient Confidentiality

We need to create that uniform data set while maintaining a very high level of patient confidentiality. The issue of patient confidentiality is an important one that needs to be handled extremely well. Patients have a high level of concern about whether or not their data will be both used appropriately and completely protected.

Interestingly, from the perspective of health care providers and payers, there really isn't an issue about whether or not individual payers should actually have that kind of patient-specific data in their computers. Why? Because that particular patient-specific part of the data storage process is in fact not at all new. It's how claims-based medical data has always been stored—by payer. All payers already have that specific full array of claims-based data about each patient in their computers now. Payers have had that data either in paper files or on their own computers for decades. Remember, payers need that information to pay claims. Insurers, health plans, and government agencies cannot and could not in fact function as payers without that data. All payers have it now.

Some consumers, however, may not realize that fact to be true. I've heard some people talk about the idea of claims payment entities having access to care-related data as though it were a new development. It is not. All payers have that data now. As patients, we get copies of our own claim forms all the time, but most of us never really look at them. Take a look at a sample claim form and see how much rich information is available on it. This is the information payers keep about each patient now.

What's new is the idea of individual health plans, insurers, and government payers making that claims-based data available back to both the patient and the patient's caregivers as an assist to the care delivery process. What is also new is the idea that the data might be aggregated—brought together in ways that protect patient confidentiality to track overall provider performance for all of their patients, regardless of which payer paid each patient's claims. Aggregate data sharing doesn't actually violate patient confidentiality if it is done right, but it is entirely new to share that data at all. So the new confidentiality issues relate to how and when claims-based data is shared—not whether health plans or other payers can or should compile it. That issue of payers actually compiling it and storing it has already been resolved. The new key issue to be resolved at this point is how to guarantee that only patients can authorize sharing of their own specific and identifiable data about themselves with other caregivers or with other people. Confidentiality at the individual patient level is a value that we should not violate in America. Compiling aggregate data that doesn't violate confidentiality for the patient but identifies overall performance patterns for the care providers is a new market value that we need to protect and support in order to achieve real reform.

Data Transferability

The details of how we actually aggregate performance data across communities have not yet been entirely worked out. Having common claims-system definitions and transferable data is essential if we want to use an electronic database to improve care and to track provider performance. We simply can't get needed levels of comparability and care process management without the context of a common data set. So we need to get agreement on those data transferability issues as soon as possible. A number of credible people and organizations are already dealing with that issue. I expect an appropriate level of agreement to happen on those issues in 2007. The American Association of Health Insurance Plans, the Blue Cross and Blue Shield Association, and the leaders of Medicare are all working to get these issues resolved.

So what should be done with that new electronic claims payment–based data set? The first priority should be to use the data to help individual patients. That claims-based electronic data set can and should be designed and formatted to produce a computerized personal health record—or PHR—for each patient. The PHR should contain electronically available information that each patient can use to keep track of his or her own care. Each patient, regardless of payer—private or public—should be entitled in a secure and confidential way to receive his own personal PHR hard-copy paper printout or electronic link to a Web version of their own electronic PHR database. That personal health record data set for each patient should show all care received by that patient, all prescriptions paid for, all tests given, all diagnoses made, and all providers who delivered care to each person as a patient. The information should be in an easy-to-use format and available to each patient on demand, either electronically or on paper. Patients should also be able to use the PHR to give their various physicians access to current information about the care being given to each patient by other physicians.

Since, as I noted earlier, people change insurance plans with some regularity, it will be important for the PHR data to be easily moved from payer to payer at the patient's request to maintain continuity of historical data. That PHR information could be used in multiple ways by patients, physicians, hospitals, and care systems to improve care. That payer-based electronic database could track far better than the current nonsystem of incomplete data sets based on paper medical files whether or not individual children have received their immunizations, for example. The data need to be both transferable between payers and then actually transferred, so if an individual child had Medicaid coverage for a while and then had private coverage for a while and also moved from one community to another, our caregivers and our community health people could still make sure that all immunizations happened for that child and that asthma care for that child was also both timely and complete. Almost fifty developing nations have higher immunization rates for preventable childhood diseases than we do,[4] in large part because we simply do not and cannot keep track very well of who has actually been immunized. (In a lot of other countries, almost every child naturally has a single medical record because local children get all care from one local provider and the complete relevant records therefore are naturally located in the hands of a single local care system and in the records of a single governmental payer. So everyone in those countries can tell from each child's single-provider record who has not yet been immunized.)

We don't have to have a single payer or a community-based single local provider to do that record keeping for each child in the United States. We can instead create a "virtual" equivalent of that process by using a single, claims payment–based data process to record all care. We could get longitudinal duty from an electronic, fully transferable personal health record–based system that creates an aggregate database for each community as well as each payer—so we could finally end the embarrassment of the United States of America having lower immunization levels than four dozen developing nations.

As I noted earlier, this will take work. To achieve real care tracking usefulness, the electronic data need to be uniform and transferable from payer to payer. They need to be built around common definitions and common codes. That work is underway.

We have already moved to common diagnosis and procedure codes across all payers. Federal standards set by the Health Insurance Portability and Accountability Act of 1996 (HIPAA) have set up consistent processes for electronic claims submission from care providers to payers.[5] So we have common codes and common data flow processes already in place. Those were major steps in the right direction. Moving now to a single provider code will almost complete that database support and creation process.

New processes will need to be created and implemented that will allow for the clean transfer of that standardized data from payer to payer as patients change their insurance vendor. Those are not unattainable market expectations or requirements. Other industries—like the airlines and banks—have already met similar challenges. It's hard to imagine an airline industry returning to paper tickets or a banking industry with only paper-based access to people's money. It's time for health care to develop similar capabilities. If the payer industry can't quickly come up with a voluntary process to get that job of transfer standardization done, it could and should be mandated by the government. Banks somehow managed to create a very workable voluntary data flow standard. So did airlines. Health care payers need to do similar work. If payers can't achieve the same data transferability goal relatively soon, the government should set those standards for everyone.

The good news is this is all very doable work.

Patients Benefit Directly from the Personal Health Record

The electronic data available now from payer computer files is pretty comprehensive. It has a wide range of possible uses. As we think about how to reform health care in this country, we need to think about how best to use that data flow. There are a lot of potentially wonderful uses. We already discussed the way a PHR could help us track a child's immunization history. In general the paper medical record database also doesn't lend itself to care protocol follow-up. The paper record is pretty much useless as a tool to track whether or not a particular patient has or has not received an appropriate medication for her illness—both because the piece of paper is inert and because for a great many patients there is no easy way to tell which provider we need to track for each individual patient. A paper medical record data infrastructure is also incapable of tracking at a broad level whether patients across a given community are getting needed care.

A child with asthma, for example, might see a pediatrician in one clinic, an urgent care doctor at a hospital, and a family practitioner in his neighborhood. As noted earlier, asthma has reached epidemic proportions among our young people. It's very often treated inadequately, and that inadequacy is particularly extreme among our minority populations.[6] So knowing whether or not each of our young asthma patients is getting appropriate treatment is a potential community health benefit. So is knowing that a percentage of all patients are or are not getting appropriate asthma care. Payer-level data is the only aggregated data source that can give us that information before everyone has an EMR available.

As we go forward to create overall computerized patient record databases by community, we also will be able to use the total database created by all local PHR files to see, for the first time ever in the history of American health care, how well various care providers do in meeting patient needs. It won't be a perfect process, but it will be very useful. In a fully computerized payment-based data set, we could run a screen for all patients with an asthma diagnosis and we could check to see (1) what asthma medications were prescribed, (2) what prescriptions were actually filled, (3) what levels of asthmas crisis (such as emergency room visits) existed, and (4) what follow-up care was done.

Once this patient population begins receiving proper treatment, the rate of painful, life-threatening asthma crisis could and should be reduced by nearly 80 percent from poorly treated levels.[7] That's a massive difference in the quality of life for those kids and their families. It's far better care than far too many kids are getting now. We really cannot improve that care in any consistent or systematic way without data, and we can't get the needed database to exist without a computer. Only a computerized database can help us figure out who is getting needed care and who is not.

Measuring Provider Performance

There are people who will be very nervous, if not completely opposed, to the creation of that provider performance database. Providers may not want to be measured. There will be patients concerned about potential personal confidentiality issues. There will be caregivers who argue that we can somehow improve care without having either available electronic data or ongoing performance measurement and performance transparency. A number of people hold those positions now with great passion. But they don't offer any other possible pathways to better, more accountable care.

Think of the practical, real-world alternatives to the electronic database. How else could we get the comparative data that is needed to improve care? We could, I suppose, skip the computers and hire a lot of people to do manual audits of a huge number of paper medical records scattered across multiple physician offices. The logistics of that approach are obviously problematic. Think about the actual steps we would have to take to gather that data. If we decided to send nurse researchers into each provider's office in any given community to dig through and evaluate the paper files for each kid (maybe three or four separate files if a kid goes to multiple caregivers), the likelihood of any particular community-wide asthma care monitoring process ever happening in any current or useful way is close to zero. Less than zero. A manual, paper-based monitoring process for asthma care would be cumbersome, inaccurate, inefficient, unaffordably expensive, inevitably incomplete, and constantly out of date. It would produce no current data that we can use to continuously improve care. By contrast, running a simple computer scan electronically through a combined, standardized, community-aggregated, personal health record commonly formatted database to look at that same data about asthma care could be simple, clean, easy, inexpensive, comprehensive, and pretty much entirely current. That would be useful data. Data that we could use to improve care.

The jury is in. If we are going to systematically improve care and recognize when care is not being delivered at acceptable levels, we need real, current, and appropriate data. The best source of that data is the fully automated electronic medical record. But that EMR-based information won't be available in most care settings for a while. In the meantime, if we want reform to happen now, we need to work with the best data we have—and the fastest and most complete source of available and usable care-based data is the current computerized insurer or payer claims filing database.

EMR Versus PHR

So if all of that information is available from the payers claims payment database, you might ask why we need an automated medical record as the next step for care improvement. Why can't we just stop with the PHR data? Let me offer a couple of thoughts on that point. The EMR is a lot more complete than a PHR and is a more directly effective care support tool.

- An EMR will have the exact prescription drug dosage and level for each patient. A PHR database may have only the name of the drug.
- Actual X-rays and scans can be embedded in a true EMR system. A PHR will just tell us the test was done and won't list the results, much less interpret them.
- The EMR will include the doctor's actual notes from each visit. The PHR will tell us only that a doctor saw a patient.
- A really good EMR will also have embedded in it an interactive advisory system that lets doctors communicate with each other as consultants. The system not only identifies that lab tests were done—it tells the results of the tests and even offers advice about how to use and interpret those results. A PHR can't do those functions.
- An EMR can have protocols embedded in it, which are useful to the doctor at the point of care. A PHR would need to have data run through an algorithm program, with advice often given after the office visit, if at all.

The EMR is a much more useful clinical tool. An EMR level of information is also the gold standard for medical review, research, and care improvement. PHR data will be very useful for research purposes, but not as useful as EMR data.

The claims-based PHR data set will, however, have very usable information. It will have diagnosis information, and it will identify care procedures by care provider. The diagnosis information will not be as complete as an EMR, but they will be sufficient to be useful. For people with diabetes, the claims-based system can track whether or not a blood sugar test was done—even though the specific results of that test may not be available at the central data level. Likewise, for people with asthma, the claims received file will show that a prescription was actually filled, but it won't show whether an unfilled prescription existed and it won't show medical notes about each patient's individual care plan.

There's also a timeliness issue. The data in a fully electronic health record tends to be current up to the minute—with updates going into the computer while the patient is actually receiving care. A claims-based system is a bit less current, with information available only after the care provider has filed a claim for payment and the claim has been processed. That used to take up to ninety days. But that situation is also changing quickly. Three quarters of all claims are now filed electronically; 30 percent of these are now submitted within a week of the service date.[8] That level of performance will continue to improve. I predict that within a couple of years, 90 percent of claims will be filed electronically within a week of the care being delivered. The other 10 percent will relate to "out of area" and emergency care needs. Pharmacy information is now often available to the payment process in real time from those pharmacies that are already electronically connected to the payer.[9] Electronic claims submission from both physicians and hospitals is the other current technology breakthrough that makes the PHR a more viable care monitoring and care support tool than it was even two years ago. I suspect that most states and most payers will mandate electronic submission of claims fairly soon.

But a pure EMR still has data much sooner—in microseconds, when the physician and hospital are connected to the EMR system. So the movement toward EMR implementation is still the right strategy. It needs to be encouraged and strongly supported.

At this stage of the game, however, to move the ball forward quickly to achieve the first levels of American health care reform,

PHR data should be good enough to begin the process. Very few people have fully appreciated yet how much short-term value this new claims-based database can add. And it's hard to overstate how important the new single provider code requirement has been to this future database.

As I noted earlier, we at Kaiser Permanente are putting in place what may well be the world's most complete electronic health record system. We're spending literally billions of dollars to do that because we believe in the full capability of that fully electronic data approach with a passion. But we know that it will take most other American caregivers and payers a bit longer to install comparable systems. So when I say that it's time for the nation as a whole to start using a partial claim-based PHR system to get the quality ball rolling, you can know that I'm not saying it to cover up an inability on our part to go the full route. We are going the full route.

At Kaiser Permanente, we are doing the whole boat electronic medical record and caregiver support system as a total package because we can. But we also know that when highly credible studies show that Americans with diabetes now receive less than half of recommended care,[10] a quickly implemented claims-based, community-centered electronic information data system could allow the status of each person with diabetes in a given community to be tracked and observed as early as next year relative to whether or not they are receiving basic blood tests, eye tests, foot status tests, and so on. That is far better than waiting five to ten years for most providers to finally glean that same information from their own mutually linked, totally automated, electronic medical record. Let's get some basic fixes in place now and not wait for five to ten years to start that electronic care support agenda.

Disease Registries Add Value

Those short-term basic data use fixes should include support for another extremely important electronic provider support tool—disease registries. Disease registries are a special set of systems that focus on patients with a given disease, such as diabetes. The registries create a special computerized database for patients with the targeted diseases. The computer registry system is fed data by the caregiver taking care of these patients. The registry creates prompts and reminders to the caregivers about best care for these patients. Reminders are very effective. One study showed that if doctors received just one simple reminder about best practices for patients with high cholesterol, they are 13 percent more likely to prescribed recommended medications, and their patients end up with a cholesterol level that is on average 19 points lower.[11] A registry that provides repeated prompts and reminders can increase consistency to levels far beyond those numbers. The key is to focus the needs of each patient and to remind the relevant doctors what those needs are.

A well-designed and -managed disease registry can perform many of the features of an electronic health record, including tracking patient lab values and medications. Until the full EMR is in place, a very good care model can be to use the PHR database to identify patients who should be in the disease registry for a given provider, and then use the more fully interactive disease registry to supply care reminders to caregivers and patients. The PHR can also help track the performance of a given disease registry for these patients. We need to strongly encourage the use of registries for many care settings, particularly those settings that aren't able or ready to put a full EMR in place.

Disease registries initially focused on just one disease. That, however, is a significant design flaw, since most of our highest-cost patients have comorbidities. It's not an efficient use of resources to have a person in three separate registries, so the newest generation of registries is being developed to deal with comorbidities. It's a far better and more logical model.

If we are going to systematically reform and improve health care in this country, we need data registries to help us track and care for chronic disease. We need an appropriate intervention from someone in health care for the relevant caregivers for any kids who are not receiving adequate asthma care. And ideally, we need both communitywide score cards and provider-specific score cards on issues like asthma care, so buyers can choose providers wisely. I'll suggest below how that might be done.

Complete Data Will Require Universal Coverage

To make the full data accountability process work at optimal levels, we also need all of those kids to have either public or private health insurance coverage. It's particularly hard to get data for uninsured people. Universal coverage is covered in Chapter Eleven of this book. As I noted earlier, the PHR claims database exists only because providers must send in relevant information in order to get paid. Logic tells us that only insured people have claims. So only insured people are in that current electronic database. Providers obviously do not send in detailed claims filing data today to any payer or nonpayer for uninsured people, so no electronic database exists anywhere today relative to their care.

That means we have a very big hole in the data bucket about the total care delivered in a community, because data from the uninsured people would not be on any computer. Introducing universal coverage as outlined in this book would solve that problem by creating a universal database about everyone's care that could and will be invaluable for both public heath data and care improvement data.

Providers Need Current Information About Best Science and Best Care

One other major reason for us to create a uniform care database and electronic communication tool that has the potential to reach out to all caregivers is the fact that the care delivery nonsystem in this country currently has an amazingly slow uptake on using new technology and approaches. I mentioned earlier that most of health care does not do systematic quality improvement. Health care also does not do rapid quality improvement. The Institute of Medicine noted that it takes seventeen years before a proven new technique becomes the standard of care in a given medical specialty.[12] As one example study showed us, even fourteen years after a particular type of medication was proven effective in treating high blood pressure, only 35 percent of people with hypertension were taking it.[13]

People from other industries who are used to six-month or shorter copycat innovation cycles are often surprised—even stunned—by the slow rate of uptake in health care for new and improved approaches.[14] Slow uptake will always be true to some degree in health care, because the stakes are so high for bad decisions. Human lives are at stake. "Defective" care can be dangerous to your health. Health care professionals are naturally very cautious about adopting any new approaches to patient treatment. That caution isn't all bad. It actually makes a lot of sense for health care to move more slowly on a lot of fronts relative to using new care. Why? Experience. The history of medical science has more than enough instances of failed new developments relative to treatment approaches that seemed in their early stages to be highly promising and later turned out to be totally wrong, even harmful.

For example, in spite of the normal caution of the medical profession, some real mistakes have been made when providers move too quickly. The use of autologous bone marrow transplants for women with breast cancer turned out to be a damaging medical fad based on insubstantial data. Women who received those particular transplants endured a far more painful treatment approach but lived no longer than women who got conventional chemotherapy.[15] The extensive use of hormone replacement therapy for menopausal women and the use of phen-fen for weight loss were equally inaccurate and ultimately dangerous medical changes that rolled out with great speed to a lot of people, to everyone's later regret.[16] So physician caution about rapid changes in practice or theory can be absolutely the right approach a very large percentage of the time.

If every potential "miracle" treatment that was temporarily profiled in the high-visibility popular press later turned out to actually have the hoped-for miraculous result, then current levels of medical caution could be more legitimately criticized. That kind of truly miraculous outcome, however, is more often the exception than the rule. As patients, we do not want our caregivers to be subject to the whims of the moment or heavily influenced by the wishes, hopes, and sometimes dramatic writings of the popular press in selecting treatment options for our own serious medical conditions. So medical caution can be a very good thing.

But medical caution can also be less than optimal, when perfectly good treatments are not picked up and used by caregivers in a relatively current time frame. The current approaches to adopting new solid science and timely improved care approaches are often too slow. A seventeen-year delay in implementing new treatments—as the IOM reported—is not even relatively current. So a better answer must be found. We need at least a middle ground for American health care. We should hold ourselves to a higher standard for the timely and effective rollout of new approaches that have been proven to work.

As I noted, many of the reasons for the delay in adopting new approaches make sense, but that doesn't mean we should accept the status quo timetable as entirely acceptable. We need to get new, well-tested approaches to the caregivers and, through the caregivers, to the patients more quickly than we do now.

If we are going to systematically improve care and move to a situation where Americans receive appropriate care more than half the time, we need to rethink how we communicate well-documented care advances to both patients and caregivers. Trying to communicate new science and new developments in care through a paper-dependent process has been an obvious failure—a logistical nightmare. Electronic communications will, I'm sure, end up being the key to significantly improving that process. Also, when patients have easy access to their own PHR, they will have more control over their care, and they will have new tools to use to check on the Internet to see if they are in fact getting the most current levels of care. That is a good thing. When patients become more demanding consumers of health care, health care providers will have to provide higher quality care and providers will need to keep up. That's a version of "good information" supply and demand. It's how the market works when it works well.

Patients already are taking some responsibility for their own care by using the Internet. Eighty percent of adult Internet users already go online to learn more about their health and their possible care.[17] That Internet-based approach will have a major new dimension when PHR data is available to all patients. An industry of Internet care consultants will, I expect, ultimately emerge to give patients "virtual specialty consults" based on their health record and current diagnosis. Patients will send their current PHR data and current diagnosis information electronically to what will be judged by patients as seemingly credible Internet physician consults. Whole new levels of care science will be made available to patients at a far faster pace through that process when it functions well.

Payers Can Help Disseminate New Information

Payers can also play an important role in getting new and relevant care information directly to caregivers and patients. Right now, as I write this, there is a new test being proposed for use in emergency rooms to see if a patient with chest pain is actually having a heart attack.[18] The new test will take two hours and cost perhaps a few hundred dollars. The old approach was to hospitalize the patient temporarily to verify or rule out a heart attack for those same patients. The old approach typically takes about twenty-four hours and costs up to $10,000 under our current payment system. So if the new brief approach actually turns out to work, what will happen under our current payment system? Will anything change relative to health care delivery and health care costs for that particular situation?

Maybe not. At least for a long while. Remember, it takes an average of five years for half of the practitioners in a given specialty to use a new and better technology, and seventeen years before it becomes the norm.

In a number of cases, I've seen the process in health care run a bit faster when the new technology is more profitable for the caregivers. In this case, however, the new process is probably less profitable for the hospitals, so there is no obvious financial incentive for most hospitals to turn twenty-four hours of relatively easy revenue into a mere two hours of billable time for large numbers of their patients.

So what should happen at this point if the health care delivery system were functioning at more cost-efficient levels? Let's assume that after study we learn that the new approach to diagnosing heart attacks actually does work better and is cheaper. Caregivers might not have an incentive to change the way things are, but insurers and other payers could have a powerful impact on the speed of roll-out for the new procedure. A uniform claims-based database on all patients could help show the payers which hospitals are using the new test and which hospitals and care teams are still using only the old $10,000 approach. Assuming that the new test is in fact both safe and accurate, buyers and payers could work directly with each reluctant caregiver to apply pressure to use the new and better approach. Payers like Medicare could simply decide to pay for the new test rather than the old approach. Provider behavior changes somewhat slowly when science is the only external input, and those same behavior changes can happen much more quickly when direct cash flow is also involved.

Some providers would probably deeply resent a new payment approach for that particular test. But they are unlikely to completely ignore the new payment approach if their new standard payment for those "rule-out" patients became based on the new low-cost methodology, rather than the old care approach.

That, however, is a heavy-handed way to effect change. An alternative would be to clearly communicate the new science electronically to all appropriate caregivers. The payer's data system itself could also be used to get new and valid scientific information about the new technology to all relevant care delivery providers if payers decide to add that important functionality to the services they provide.

We are on the very edge of using the Internet to improve care in a great many ways, both with individual patients and with caregivers. If major payers used the Internet to send information about the new test to each caregiver who is still using the old approach, then the caregiver would not need to wait years to attend a seminar to learn the new technique.

Likewise, the Internet can and should be used to help providers of care keep up with the best new asthma drugs, the best heart attack diagnostic tests, and the best new knee surgery prosthetics. Someone has to do that information dissemination work, or it will not get done. A more current set of outcomes-based information can be communicated to individual caregivers in a far more systematic way if that communication process becomes an assigned role done on behalf of patients and buyers by various health plans or benefit administrators using the linkages already created by the payment process. Infrastructure reform is needed. We need a market model that will cause infrastructure reform to happen.

The next three chapters of this book talk about alternative new market approaches that would create a new value-linked business model for health care. One key to that process will be getting current information about best care to caregivers in a far more systematic way.

Two Hundred to Thirty Thousand

One final point on that issue. We all need to recognize exactly why it is not an easy thing for care providers to stay current on medical science. In 1975, there were only 200 medical clinical trials published. A doctor could almost read 200 clinical trials each year. Marcus Welby might have known everything there was to know about medicine in 1975. A decade later, in 1985, that number had climbed to 2,000 published trials. A physician might keep up with 200. It's a lot harder to keep up with 2,000 studies. By 1995, that number had jumped to 10,000 articles—all credible pieces published in formal refereed journals. Ten thousand articles are even harder to read. By 2005, the number had jumped to 30,000 articles. That's a lot of science, as Figure 3.1 graphically demonstrates. Having 30,000 clinical trials done and published instead of just 200 is actually very good news for the patients, but in the real world, it is just a bit difficult for an individual caregiver whose day job is treating a full schedule of patients to keep up. We now need very well-designed tools to support the caregivers in keeping up. These tools needs to involve the computer, or they will be totally unworkable.

That "keeping up" work needs to be done by someone who does it for a living, if it is to be done at all. Amazingly, under the current approach, no one is accountable for sharing and disseminating that information to our physicians and other caregivers. Having no one

Figure 3.1. Published Clinical Trials, 1975–2005.

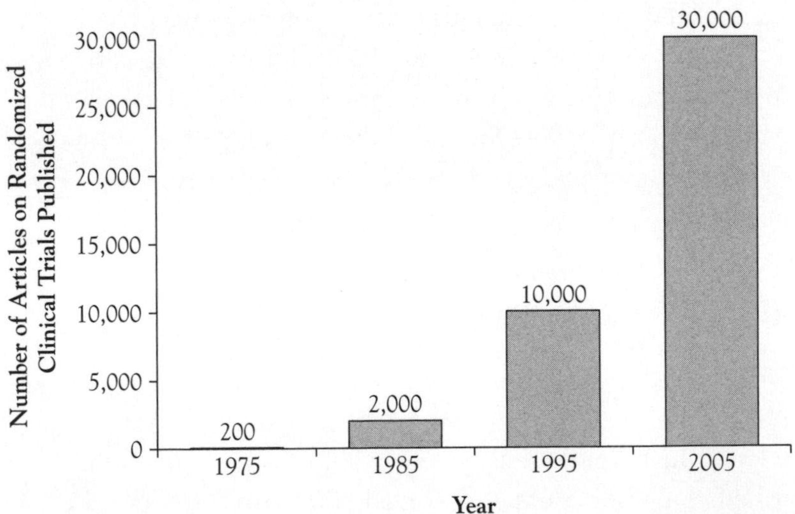

Sources: M. R. Chassin, "Is Health Care Ready for Six Sigma Quality?" *Milbank Quarterly*, 1998, 76(4), 565–591; R. Rubin, "In Medicine, Evidence Can Be Confusing." *USA Today*, Oct. 16, 2006.

accountable for that information flow to providers obviously is a massively flawed approach, and we've seen the results.

Health Care Needs a New Market Model

Health care reform needs to be done in the context of a systems-based strategy and a new market model. American health care will not evolve into a system with a high level of data accuracy and information currency on its own. The evolution of health care into a new, more accountable market model needs to be carefully guided, with the same level of energy and attention that buyers now apply to the specifications they create every day for hubcaps or computer cards. Buyers don't say, "Send me any hubcaps you have available." They specify every detailed aspect of the hubcaps they are buying. There's no reason that the health care purchasing process should end up at a lower level of buyer competency. Buyers spend a lot more money on health care than they do on hubcaps—even auto manufacturers do. The key will be to help the buyers figure out exactly what those care purchase specifications should be.

To start the whole process out, a first goal of the new purchasing model should be a data-rich environment, with better research, improved performance, and better choices. Consumers should be able to make real choices about both caregivers and care because comparative data will be available about each possible choice. Caregivers themselves should have a data flow in place that will allow for systematic care improvement, and that can give them an initial level of badly needed feedback about care. Payers also will benefit from a uniform, aggregated, shared database. The claims-based database is a good first step in that direction.

The Culture of Health Care Needs to Evolve

It's actually hard to imagine how unsystematic and data-free most care is today and how hard the existing culture of care resists the intrusion of process-based data. People from other industries who are used to a world where data tracking and systematic thinking about process and outcomes are both normal behavior have a hard time realizing how completely inadequate the available performance database is for caregivers today. Anyone used to Six Sigma thinking or systematic CQI approaches would find health care to be incredibly rich in process improvement opportunities and poverty-stricken when it comes to actual process improvement projects, successes, and even measurement.

Please read Don Berwick's book, *Escape Fire: Designs for the Future of Health Care*.[19] Berwick is one of the gurus of American medical quality. His wife was hospitalized with a serious illness. In the book, he tells of his wife's hospital care—and reports that some of the best hospitals in America made roughly one error in her care each day. Had he, as a trained physician, not been present at her bedside, a couple of these mistakes could have cost her her life. The information flow in our current health care infrastructure was not uniform. It was not adequate. Care linkage deficiencies happened for his wife even in intensive inpatient hospital care settings. Whether or not a medication had been given was not always known. Physician instructions were not always understood. Please read that book. It's a brilliant and insightful piece of work.

Berwick argues persuasively that it is time for health care to change its culture and value systems to think systematically about improving the quality, safety, and efficiency of care. In his words, "A patient with anything but the simplest needs is traversing a very complicated system across many handoffs and locations and players. And as the machine gets more complicated, there are more ways it can break."[20] He is absolutely right. And we need to create both the tools and the cultural changes needed to make that level of reform happen.

Culture Trumps Strategy

There's an old saying in business that "culture trumps strategy." Another version of that adage says, "Culture eats strategy for lunch." In either case, the point is that inside an organization or an industry, when strategies and cultures collide, strategies do not always win. How is that issue relevant to this book?

Health care in this country has some deep-seated cultural beliefs and practices that can frankly make CQI types of thinking and decision making problematic at best, and impossible at worst, in far too many settings. Health care is an ultimate bastion of the "not invented here" approach to idea rejection. That approach is a common element in a lot of health care cultures. Other industries constantly seek out best practices, and business units steal from other sites and competitors regularly. That best practice sharing process is both a cultural value and a basic operational mode of doing business in most industries. If a manufacturer discovers that a competitor is using a new distribution process, for example, the manufacturer will often study the new process intently and they will steal, or attempt to copy, any part of the new process that seems to work particularly well.

Health care goes to an opposite extreme. The culture of health care can directly and strongly oppose shared learning at very local levels, even about common issues like chart transfer processes. The people who run one floor of a hospital often don't even want to know how the people on another floor of the same hospital handle a particular process, procedure, or problem. Take a universal task as basic as the change of the nurse shift information transfer process, for example. Hospitals are open twenty-four hours a day. So multiple shifts are needed for each work site and unit. At the end of each shift, the nurses from the prior shift take some time to brief the new set of nurses about each patient in the relevant work unit. That's a very good thing to do. It's essential for continuity of patient care. It's a job that has to be done three times a day—hopefully very well, because the quality of the information sharing affects the quality of care for each patient.

Unfortunately, that process is not always done either well or efficiently. It can take a lot of time. The communication process itself can too easily create factual errors. It's a typical type of American care linkage deficiency—one that we may more readily expect from outpatient clinical care, but one that is somehow a bit more surprising when it happens in an institution as formal and highly organized as a hospital. In the real world of American health care, each floor in a hospital is likely to have its own separate information transfer process, "invented here, by us." People in other hospitals, even in the same town, don't typically try to find out who has the best process for transitioning that information. Process improvement as a desirable cultural value doesn't show up at all on a lot of health care radar screens.

The good news is that means that a lot of low-hanging fruit currently exists in health care. When real process improvement thinking is finally introduced, and the culture of health care adapts continuous improvement as a shared value, the initial improvements can be huge—and relatively easy. For the nurse shift transfer process, for example, simply implementing an easy-to-use, standardized, well–thought out, carefully designed information checklist for use with each patient can cut the transfer time from nurse to nurse from over half an hour per shift change to under fifteen minutes while reducing communication errors about individual patients hugely.[21] Patient safety improves. Nurse efficiency improves. Care linkages improve. The nurses who are tired and worn out at the end of their shifts get to go home a bit earlier. And everyone wins.

But that isn't how most health care settings work. Setting up and refining best processes in a systematic way is a whole new operational science for most caregivers. No one is trained to do that work. No one is assigned to do that work. The culture of care resists that work. It's not a good thing.

The opportunities are everywhere. Setting up a simple presurgery safety checklist for surgery teams, similar to the one used by airline pilots before takeoff, seems like elementary basic common sense from the perspective of a full-blown CQI culture—particularly when that kind of organized information-sharing process can reduce errors like wrong-site surgery to close to zero.[22] But that same type of process-based thinking can be seen as a radical and unwelcome intrusion into the personal and professional prerogatives of surgery unit leaders from another existing cultural perspective. Brave people in health care management are actually often afraid to even marginally intrude into that cultural minefield. Health care professionals who know how to significantly improve both safety and efficiency sometimes hesitate and then choose not to even raise those basic issues in ways that might offend the hard-core believers in individual care unit autonomy. In those cases, culture wins—and the culture that wins is not one that creates improvement in the process of care. Perfectly reasonable process improvement ideas can get totally rejected by that cultural milieu. In a truly worst-case setting, they don't even get rejected. They simply never even get raised.

Why would health care leadership in various settings allow that culture of fierce resistance to standardized, optimal, consistent processes to continue?

Sometimes it's a business issue for certain types of caregivers. Hospital CEOs, for example, have often been very reluctant to raise those kinds of process improvement issues with various independent surgical groups who voluntarily bring their patients to the hospital. Those independent surgical groups are generally wooed by every hospital in town. They represent major revenue. Everyone wants their patients. So those surgical groups often expect the hospital they use to either completely meet their stated needs, demands, and cultural expectations or get out of their way. Hospital administrators in multiple settings can each very clearly describe the economic incentives they have to keep those surgical groups happy and admitting patients to their facility. Seminars are held at hospital conventions on how to attract and keep these groups. So the administrators often don't put a lot of pressure on those groups. A number of the hospital administrators that I've talked to often aren't very happy about that situation. But it's how the economics of hospital management often work.

That's actually one reason why externally imposed quality requirements can be a real blessing to many hospital leaders and to many independent hospitals. Instead of being able to make process improvement changes from within, many of these frustrated, economically challenged, and unfortunately passive hospital administrators are often delighted to use external pressures to overcome their own institution's internal cultural barriers to implementing effective process quality improvement campaigns. To succeed in changing each hospital's caregiving culture, those external pressures have to be focused on the desired results, not details of the desired process. The 100,000 Lives Campaign organized by Donald Berwick and his Institute for Healthcare Improvement (IHI) was a brilliant effort in that direction.[23] By bringing an inspired combination of external good science and high moral suasion efforts to bear simultaneously, Berwick gave hospital leaders across the country the leverage point they needed to overcome the historic status quo culture of many care sites. Hospital leaders and their enlightened physician allies were given leverage points and persuasive tools they needed to make systematic enhancements in their hospital's operational processes. The new care safety science of the 100,000 Lives Campaign wasn't actually entirely new. What was new was the moral and operational leverage created inside many hospitals by the new highly publicized external quality improvement expectations. One important result of that campaign was 122,300 lives saved as of June 14, 2006,[24] but even more important, the result was a new functional perspective in many hospital cultures about systematic improvement. It was a big step in a good direction. Millions of Americans are in Berwick's debt.

Large, multispecialty physician group practices generally face fewer cultural barriers to improving care than do care cultures that revolve around individual physician practices. Large groups have built-in peer review processes that typically are evidence-based and mitigate against excessively arbitrary decision making by any unit leaders. The Mayo Clinic, for example, has a spectacular culture of focusing on continuously improving best care.[25] Those values are deeply embedded in that culture, and they drive Mayo care decisions every single day. Mayo doctors hold each other accountable as a group and as individuals for best care. Mayo Care. But in health care settings where that peer pressure for optimal care does not exist, the local culture too often completely trumps any attempts at systematic thinking about care processes or care improvement.

This is an important issue for American health care reform. Cultures in any setting are a fabric of expectations woven from various belief system threads that embody values, rules, standards, and behaviors. Changing the culture in any setting can be done by explicitly and strategically changing a belief, a value, a rule, or a common behavior. The culture of American health care today does not include beliefs, values, or behaviors that focus on data-driven improvement processes. That needs to change. Health care needs to do a better job of both using data and thinking systematically about operational improvement. Rules and external expectations can both help. Those values about continuous improvements, systematic thinking, and use of data to help improve care tend not to be embedded in the current provider culture in most care settings.

So what can be done to change that situation? It would be cumbersome, excessively bureaucratic, relatively inflexible, generally inadequate, and sometimes entirely dysfunctional to have the new best practice operational guidelines and processes in those areas imposed by external forces. For example, it would not be optimal to have a single, uniform national presurgery checklist process or a statewide nurse shift transition process that was externally mandated for use by all caregivers. Those processes would be too rigid and often not amenable to continuous enhancement and improvement. However, it is perfectly reasonable to use both market forces and moral suasion to incent and inspire caregivers to use their own creativity and problem-solving skills to fix the major operational issues that obviously exist in far too many settings. It is also perfectly reasonable for the various regulators and certification processes to ask for evidence that those issues are being addressed. As one example, it would be a very good thing for hospital accreditation processes to include a requirement that hospitals all implement programs to identify, measure, and verifiably fix those kinds of communication and linkage problems. We are beginning to see some thinking in those directions. It would also be workable to introduce external measurement requirements of the communication errors that happen at shift transitions in hospitals or the errors that happen in surgical units during surgery as the result of inadequate or inconsistent transmission of needed information. To achieve competitive performance and quality improvement, such measurements should be required—and some are long overdue. Such measurements can be imposed externally and in a uniform manner, while solutions should be devised internally according to what best fits that particular institution.

From Resistance to Brilliance

My own belief is that when continuous improvement values are finally woven into the fabric of the American health care culture, our caregivers will go from resistance to brilliance, and American ingenuity will transform care in ways we can't even begin to anticipate now. When the culture and the reward system both support continuous improvements, that behavior will become the new norm for health care thinking. We are not there yet. There is no significant economic or reputational downside now for hospitals or surgical teams who have higher than average error rates in either of those processes. There is no cultural expectation that we should continuously improve our outcomes in these ways. Each unit on each floor in each surgery can invest in and insist on its own idiosyncratic, unmeasured approach because there are no consequences for either inefficiency or inaccuracy. So local unit-specific power structures and cultures prevail, and massive inconsistency results.

Process improvement happens in manufacturing both as practice and culture—not because Wal-Mart or Target designs or manages the actual manufacturing processes or micromanages actual steps involved in production—but because they clearly specify the detailed process outcomes. Very importantly, they specify the allowable error rate. The individual manufacturers then do their own thinking and their own process design work to achieve the lower error rate. The internal staff and management cultures of each manufacturer's business change to promote and favor continuous improvement values and skills as a second-level consequence of the efforts needed to reduce errors to that targeted rate.

Processes Will Improve When Targets Are Set

Health care will follow a similar path when buyer specifications are significantly improved. Processes will improve when targets are set that cannot be met without process improvement techniques. When that happens, process improvement skills will be learned, and comparative data will help caregivers improve their own performance levels on key measurements relative to other caregivers.

The intermediate steps require goals and measurements. Measurements must lead to comparisons. Comparisons must lead to consequences. Consequences will lead to behavior changes—and that will result in overall process improvement and in a culture of process improvement. None of those steps can be skipped if we really want improved care delivery. Attempting to institute consequences before we have data or attempting to do comparisons before we have measurement are obviously inadequate ways of achieving real reform.

Consequences, as outlined in Chapters Six and Seven, must be market-based and must originate from enlightened buyers—or the whole market reform process will be doomed to inadequacy as a result. Buyers must play the same role for health care that Target and Wal-Mart now play for product manufacturers: rewarding vendors that meet rigorous specifications and moving away from vendors who fail to meet those specifications.

What's Next?

So how can incentives for quality improvement be created? We need a market model that might get the job done in a relatively short period of time.

Before looking at a proposed market model, let's spend a few pages looking at the five chronic conditions that cause most of our care expenses, to see a few very basic things that we can do to bring these costs down. The next chapter is a very practical look at a few things we need to do to really improve the quality and costs of care in America.

It's not rocket science. It's just a very basic application of systems thinking to care improvement for a few conditions.

The point of discussing that specific information about those five diseases in this book is to simply show it can be done. I included the next chapter in the book to demystify the process. We have a huge financial opportunity relative to those specific patients. It's not a terribly complex set of things that we need to do. We need basic common sense and current science applied systematically to care for each of those patients. If you already know that to be true, you can skip the next chapter and go directly to the eight elements that will make health care reform possible.

But you may want to take a quick look first at the key conditions that drive most health care costs and what we can do to make care better and costs lower for the people who have those specific health conditions. Those treatment approaches are not so complex that it takes a trained medical mind to appreciate the potential for improvement. However, to be entirely transparent, I did involve a couple of trained medical minds to help me write the chapter. They have my deep gratitude.

As you read about those approaches, I suspect you'll also appreciate why some of the data tools outlined in this chapter could be better designed and more fully developed for both care improvement and real market reform.

Data is the missing ingredient. We need real data about care performance as soon as we can get it. Then we need to use that data to reform care.

Read on for some thoughts about how that might be done.

4

Basic Steps to Improve Care for Chronic Disease Patients

What can we actually do with the information that a relatively small number of patients incur most of the health care costs in America? We know who those patients are. We know exactly what care they need. We have developed excellent, though costly, care for those patients when they become acutely ill. However, we also know that if we do everything right as a care delivery infrastructure, we can intervene well before the most expensive and debilitating acute illness stages of each disease happen. By bringing together caregivers as a team to deal with both the comorbidities and the cumulative progression of these diseases, we can systematically reduce the likelihood that those patients will actually become acutely ill.

The good news is that we can, in fact, actively intervene in very effective ways with chronic care patients to prevent the onset or slow the progression of their diseases. As a result of those interventions, we can make a huge difference in both quality of life and costs of care for many people who otherwise will be our most expensive patients.

In other words, we can make a real difference as a care infrastructure in the lives and care of people with chronic disease, providing the right treatments, the right medications, the right lifestyle counseling, and the right follow-up care. But far too often that whole pattern of needed right care does not happen, and the result is far too many complications, unnecessary deterioration in people's health, and a needless decrease in the quality of many people's lives.

So what exactly should we be doing as an infrastructure of care to improve our performance for these chronic care patients? How can we systematically intervene so that our most expensive patients don't become acutely ill at all and others experience many fewer complications with their diseases? The answers to those questions are not as complex as some people might think.

I wrote this chapter to make it clear that many of the care delivery issues we are facing with regard to our highest-cost patients are not incredibly complicated, esoteric, complex medical science issues that can only be understood by fully trained subspecialty medical practitioners. The issues are pretty basic: blocking and tackling, making connections between caregivers, and creating high levels of patient understanding about their medical behaviors and their care.

The chapter will show you that there really is something very practical and doable that we can implement for the patients who incur most of our costs.

If you already know what I am talking about and have any time pressure in your life, you might find it convenient to move on now to the next chapter where I discuss the eight new developments that have made health reform care possible. If you do that, however, I'd recommend returning to this chapter at some point for a quick refresher on some basic facts and issues.

As I noted in Chapter One, most of America's health care costs come from patients with one or more chronic diseases—congestive heart failure, asthma, diabetes, coronary artery disease, and depression—and each of those five chronic diseases tends to be a progressive disease that can be impacted positively by appropriate and timely interventions. The risk factors for those diseases are well known. The protocols for slowing the progression of each disease are equally well known. The medical science is pretty clear. If patients get the right medications and medical monitoring and make the right behavioral changes, the potential to reduce complications and to improve outcomes for these diseases is substantial.

The biggest cost savings come from preventing the acute care crises and intense medical complications that evolve from these diseases. Kidney failure in the United States, for example, is most often a complication of late-stage diabetes. As many as 10 percent of people with diabetes go on to develop chronic kidney disease.[1] In more than half of new kidney failure patients—nearly a quarter million people between 2000 and 2004—diabetes is the cause of end-stage renal disease.[2] With appropriate and consistent diabetic care supported by basic patient behavioral changes, the number of kidney failures in this country could be cut by at least one third.[3] Some argue that the reduction could be even greater.

And kidney disease is not the only comorbidity with diabetes. Diabetes is also the number-one cause of new blindness and foot and leg amputations, and is the number-one comorbidity associated with death from heart failure. Each of those highly acute care crises can be significantly reduced by better early care for our diabetic patients. Go to the American Diabetes Association web site and pull up the Diabetes PhD interactive computer program based on the Kaiser Permanente Archimedes modeling program[4] to see how large the impact on diabetes can be if each patient has the right approach to both behavior change and care. The opportunity is huge. (If you are diabetic yourself, you could find the Diabetes PhD web site to be an invaluable source of learning and counsel.)

If we can encourage people to change their behavior so that they are much less likely to develop Type II (adult onset) diabetes, that would be the best outcome. That should be a major goal. But even after diabetes has been diagnosed, the current unrealized opportunities for better care and better health are enough to have a major positive potential impact on the cost of care for America.

Again, this isn't rocket science. It's the basic application of consistent, coordinated, well-designed, and strategically focused care system approaches to the needs and health status of individual patients.

Congestive Health Failure

Let's start with congestive heart failure. About five million people in the United States have congestive heart failure, and each year more than a half million people are diagnosed with it for the first time.[5] In heart failure, the heart can't pump with enough force to move blood throughout the body. Heart failure develops over time as the heart muscle grows weaker and weaker.

The major underlying causes of heart failure are coronary artery disease, high blood pressure, and diabetes.[6] It's the most common diagnosis in hospital patients aged sixty-five and older.[7] It's one of the most expensive diseases in America. Congestive heart failure can also be a very unpleasant disease. When congestive heart failure hits its most acute stage, people experience a state of intense crisis. The heartbeat isn't strong enough to keep the blood moving forward, so there is a backup of liquid. The body can retain so much fluid that people's hearts and lungs are literally drowning in their own fluids. It's a terrible situation to find yourself in. People in the middle of a congestive heart failure crisis end up in the hospital fighting for their lives, in pain, sometimes in terror. It's so bad that caregivers sometimes deliberately knock patients unconscious to facilitate the whole drainage process. It's definitely a time and situation to be avoided, if at all possible.

Fortunately for the vast majority of congestive heart failure (CHF) patients, that crisis is now generally avoidable. Avoiding crisis is not only much better for the patient, it's a lot less expensive. Inpatient hospital admissions for CHF are extremely expensive, particularly when the CHF patient is near death. Intensive care units expend a lot of resources keeping CHF patients alive. It's far better for everyone involved to avoid those crises as often as possible.

Congestive Heart Failure Treatment

So what can be done to help CHF patients avoid those costly and painful admissions? Treatment focuses on (1) relieving strain on the heart as much as possible with blood pressure reducing drugs, (2) using other medications—beta blockers—which have been shown to "calm" a failing heart and allow it to work more efficiently, and (3) in combination with reducing salt in the diet (which causes fluid retention), using diuretics or fluid pills to remove excess fluids and keep a patient as close as possible to their most functional weight.

Once a patient has been diagnosed as having CHF and has stabilized on the right doses of medicines, the patient needs to be very well educated about the early warning signs of a CHF crisis. Quick weight gain, for example, is a strong indicator of upcoming trouble. When the CHF patient starts to retain fluids, weight goes up. By monitoring his or her weight every day, the patient can get an early warning that trouble is imminent, and get immediate help either at an outpatient clinic or even in his or her own home. Usually, a brief increase in the diuretic dose will be enough to stabilize the disease.

Early treatment of these early indicators like weight gain or increasing shortness of breath means far fewer hospital admissions. However, both the patient's and the caregiver's reaction time to these indicators has to be very fast or the situation can deteriorate very quickly to the point where a life is at stake and only a hospital can provide the needed care. To insure that patients are monitored closely and get the advice and coaching they need about their disease, specialized nurses who understand heart failure well can work closely with the patient and their families, over the phone or through home visits. These "care managers" can work closely with heart failure doctors and can recognize important changes early, keep the patient connected to the doctor's care by guiding treatment changes, and prevent many serious episodes of heart failure that might otherwise lead to hospitalization.

By doing everything right in that care package, inpatient admissions for CHF patients can be reduced by 50 percent.[8] "Doing it right" requires a carefully committed team of caregivers working together on behalf of each CHF patient. To eliminate care linkage deficiencies for CHF patients, team care is needed, and the team needs to be linked together.

Most CHF patients interact with the actual care system only at a time of crisis, when the disease has already moved without intervention to an extremely acute stage.[9] They often encounter the care delivery infrastructure for the first time in the emergency room of the hospital, at a point where the hospital needs to do heroic work just to keep the patient alive.

American hospitals do great deeds at that point—miracles, really—often at great expense, and often at great emotional and physical cost to the patient.

We as a nation should find that situation unacceptable at multiple levels. We need to ensure that far fewer CHF patients reach this acute state of crisis. When we treat CHF as a chronic progressive disease instead of as an acute episode, we can greatly improve patient care. There is a lot we can do. We need to diagnose CHF earlier and then insist on best care for our CHF patients. We should ensure that each of those patients receives well-linked, team-based care directed at preventing those horrible, painful, excessively expensive medical crises, as well as mitigating the ongoing deterioration of patient health that results from the disease.

Systemness and Congestive Heart Failure

Obviously, this is a situation where "systemness" is highly relevant, even essential. Care linkage deficiencies damage CHF patients. Health care organizations with complete, well-linked care teams are the best setting for CHF patients. Where such teams don't exist, or when the patient doesn't choose that kind of care setting, the same level of inter-caregiver linkages should still be set up on a computer-linked virtual basis, with caregivers who take care of each CHF patient making sure as a virtual team that the right monitoring is being done, the right prescriptions are being filled, and that the precrisis interventions are swift and effective.

Hospitals can play a major role in that process by helping to coordinate and integrate the work of the doctors who treat CHF patients in their clinics and the doctors who admit CHF patients to their settings. Doctors who treat CHF patients can and should put together their own set of nurses and support staff to support consistent care and to contact CHF patients to determine when early interventions are needed. Without those consistent contacts and linkages, the actual number of life-threatening and extremely painful CHF crises in America is more than twice as high as it needs to be.

Keep in mind that given the way we pay American health care providers today, safely preventing a CHF crisis might generate only $200 in billable revenue for caregivers. Allowing a CHF crisis to occur for that same patient could result in $10,000 to $20,000 in billable revenue. Think about that difference: $200 versus $20,000. If you believe in using economics as a motivating factor, it's obvious that our current financial incentives for caregivers clearly are not well designed for CHF patients. I'll return to that topic in Chapter Six on the use of market forces to improve care.

If we go forward as a nation to put in place the communitywide, claims record–based PHR electronic database for each community that was outlined in the prior chapter of this book, then basic patterns of linked or unlinked care for CHF patients could be tracked by purchasers of care, payers, or various community health oversight programs. Those oversight programs—hospitals, care organizations, or health plans—could use the new electronic personal health record database as a mechanism for understanding what actually is happening for those patients.

As I'll outline in Chapter Six, buyers who don't insist on hiring some functional entity to track, monitor, influence, and reward optimal provider performance in those areas are missing a significant opportunity to be far better purchasers of care. This is the kind of high-cost, high-impact area where purchasers can and should purchase wisely. It's pretty basic stuff.

Developing expert specifications for CHF follow-up is not a difficult concept for buyers to address. It's a little like heavy equipment manufacturers expecting their parts vendors to meet minimum quality specifications for key pieces of equipment. That's almost common sense, when so many dollars are involved and the potential rewards are so high. Asking vendors to explain their CHF strategies to the buyer is not at all an unreasonable request. Asking for proof of success is also not a bad idea. A lot of money and a lot of human discomfort and pain are both at stake. It's a topic that should be on the table as a buyer expectation.

Asthma

Let's take a look at another of the five dire diseases: asthma. Asthma is the fastest growing disease in America for kids. Over the last twenty years, its prevalence in children and teens has nearly doubled, to the point where more than six million children suffer from asthma today.[10] The burden of asthma isn't evenly distributed either, as Figure 4.1 demonstrates.

No one is quite sure why asthma is growing so rapidly, but it's exploding for both kids and adults. Asthma accounts for over two million emergency room visits, 500,000 hospital stays, and 5,000 deaths every year.[11] That makes it one of the five chronic diseases that create the bulk of our health care costs.

Hospitalizations for asthma can be extremely expensive. Asthma can also cost society in other ways. Asthma is a disease that undermines a person's health and personal functionality on an almost constant basis. People miss school and work. In 2004, more than fourteen million days of school and work were lost due to asthma.[12] Asthma patients function poorly on a regular basis, and people and

Figure 4.1. Prevalence of Asthma Among White and Black Americans, 2001 and 2004.

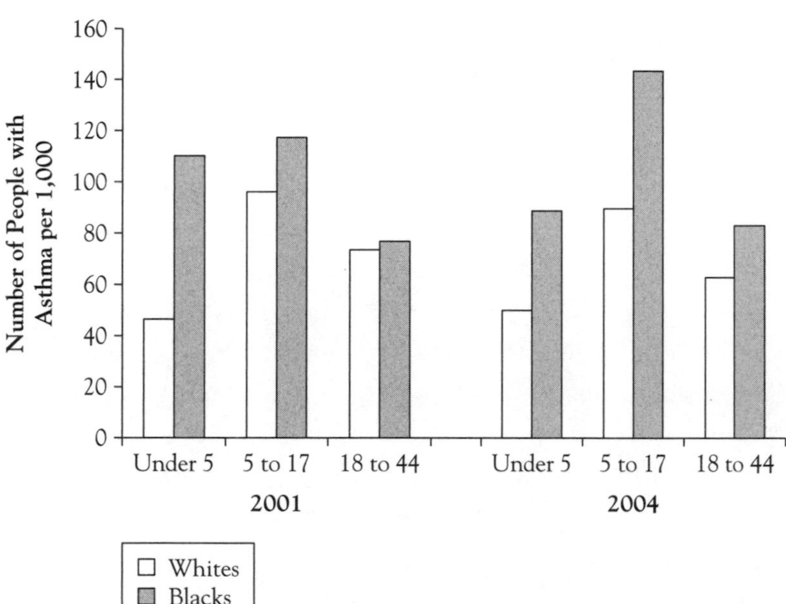

Source: American Lung Association, "Trends in Asthma Morbidity and Mortality 2006," July 2006, table 9.

their families experience a really lousy quality of life with some levels of chronic asthma symptoms.

Human Cost

As with congestive heart failure, there is a lot more than money at stake here. The direct human cost of asthma should not be underestimated. Like CHF, asthma has its terrible times of crisis. When someone experiences an acute asthma attack, it can be terrifying. In a mild attack, breathing becomes difficult and may be painful. In a severe attack, it's almost impossible to breathe. Left untreated, people die.

In an asthma attack, breathing tubes in the lungs become narrowed and obstructed. This happens because patients with asthma have sensitive inflammatory cells within the lining of their breathing tubes that react in a harmful way to things in the air like pollen, dust, and animal dander. While we all have these inflammatory cells and they protect us from infections and other inhaled threats, in patients with asthma they are hypersensitive. They react to triggers, swelling the lining of the breathing tubes, secreting mucous into the middle of the tubes, and tightening small muscles that surround parts of the breathing tubes. The breathing tubes become very narrow, and the patient feels like he or she is breathing through a smaller and smaller straw. The narrowed and inflamed tubes and secretions also lead to wheezing and coughing, causing more misery.

In an acute crisis-level attack, emergency room caregivers respond by giving the patient extra oxygen to inhale, reducing some of the strain on the lungs, and using inhaled and intravenous medicines to expand the narrowed airways. Finally, powerful anti-inflammatory medicines called glucocorticoids are given to counteract the inflammation that started the attack. While acute treatment usually reverses an acute asthma attack, it has side effects, is frightening and expensive, and can almost always be avoided with good, comprehensive, and coordinated asthma care.

Emergency room (ER) visits are not only expensive; they are also generally not a particularly pleasant experience. ERs tend to be staffed by wonderful people doing a lot of great work in a crisis mode to save lives and help people recover from health emergencies. ER patients are usually there because they are in trouble. So ERs tend to be full of people in crisis—including patients who may have been stabbed, are having a heart attack, propping up a broken limb, throwing up, or gasping painfully for breath. Simply being in the ER space as a patient can be an unpleasant and unforgettable experience for both the patient and his or her friends and family, even when the patient does badly need the ER care.

The care in the ER itself is usually superb, but the staff in many ERs tend to be overworked and sometimes close to overwhelmed. If you want to look at the bigger picture for ERs, whenever the ER staff in an institution is already overworked, any strategy that cuts their workload by reducing the actual number of people in crisis is good for the caregivers and other patients as well.

So any care intervention process that eliminates the need for otherwise healthy asthmatics to use an ER has real merit on several levels—for payers, for caregivers, and especially for patients.

Early Interventions

Asthma is a progressive chronic disease like congestive heart failure that lends itself to early interventions. People with asthma need to be individually trained to recognize early that an attack is coming on, and each patient needs to be trained and equipped to intervene directly to stop that attack. Interventions work.

In a solid treatment regimen, a patient with frequent asthma would take anti-inflammatory medications to keep oversensitive inflammatory cells under control. These medications can be taken using an inhaler, which is a mechanical device patients use to pump medications into their own lungs. By delivering these "preventer" medications directly to the underlying problem area, inhalers minimize the side effects of these powerful medicines.

In a less severe attack, patients can also self-medicate with an additional inhaler containing "reverser" medications, such as albuterol, to help dilate breathing tubes. These reverser medications are used to supplement the more powerful preventer medications, but are inadequate for moderate to severe asthma, the type that leads to severe attacks.

Again, like CHF, an absolute, very basic key to success is doing the right thing at the right time for each patient and doing it well very quickly. Once the optimal moment for intervention passes, the likelihood of a hospitalization for the asthma patient increases sharply—at least for an emergency room visit and related interventions.

Prevention of those hospital care encounters involves careful patient education, written action plans, reminders, and team-based care so the patient can detect symptoms early and take steps to stop the asthma attacks early. School-based interventions for children and teens with asthma are common.[13] In one innovative approach, teens receive reminders on cell phones to take their medications.[14] Ideally, each asthma patient needs to be ready to respond effectively to the early symptoms that indicate a progression of their disease. A missed opportunity to use an appropriate inhaler early in a deteriorating situation can result all too quickly in a major asthma crisis and in an unpleasant and very expensive emergency room visit.

Six Sigma Care

Again, asthma is an area of great opportunity for this country. We often do a very incomplete job of asthma care in America.[15] Most caregivers who treat asthma patients do not work as a strategically linked team both with other caregivers and with the patient to respond to crisis or to prevent future occurrences of the disease.

Too many people, including people with asthma, assume prevention isn't possible. They assume they have to live with acute attacks. The truth is, prevention is often very possible. But teaching people how to achieve prevention will typically not happen in ER-based care settings, where the staff is too busy to deal with proactive care issues.

In addition, the ER staff generally does not have time to deal with asthma triggers. There are a lot of potential external triggers for asthma attacks. A really well-designed patient-focused care system will systematically explore, discover, and then mitigate the individual triggers for each patient. Key questions need to be regularly asked and answered. Are allergies involved? Is there mold in the patient's environment? Second-hand smoke? First-hand smoke?

Again, think about how we would treat asthma from a Six Sigma or continuous quality improvement perspective. Think systematically. We'd ask: What is the process of events, and what are the triggers that lead to this patient's asthma attacks? We know from research data that many asthma attacks have very specific external triggers.[16] A systematic approach aimed at preventing or reducing the number of asthma attacks for each patient would consistently seek out and then use that information for each patient, instead of just treating the patient in the ER as a fee-for-service reimbursed incident of care after yet another unexplained, crisis-level asthma attack occurred.

The vast majority of asthma attacks can be prevented when patient-specific triggers are identified.[17] A health care system aiming for Six Sigma–like results would always ask a few key questions about those triggers. Always.

Do you, as a purchaser of health care or health coverage, know whether or not those questions are being either asked or answered in the asthma care approach you pay for? Do you, as an asthma patient, know whether or not your doctor is systematically looking for causation? Do you, as a patient, know whether or not the drugs being prescribed for your asthma control are the most appropriate drugs? Do you know what early symptoms of an asthma attack look like—and do you have a plan that you understand that helps you know when and how to take the right medication in the right quantities to stop an attack before it worsens? Written action plans are key to successful self-management.[18]

Creating the Best Program

Caregivers optimally need to educate each and every patient on both asthma triggers and effective responses to early symptoms. Don't think of care as being just the direct encounter that occurs in an exam room, emergency room, or hospital room after the crisis has begun. Think literally outside those physical treatment site boxes.

Education can be a key treatment step for asthma patients.

Some of the best asthma patient education programs use group sessions of similar patients—teenagers, for example—who can help each other by sharing response strategies and offering mutual encouragement about actively and proactively controlling the negative impact of the disease. Having groups of teenagers with asthma explain to each other how they deal with asthma as a life factor and how they react to early asthma symptoms in various real-world settings can all by itself cut the number of future asthma crises.

Again, as with CHF, the best asthma programs can have more than a 75 percent reduction in the incidence of those painful, life-threatening, and extremely expensive crisis events.[19] If the care system meets Six Sigma consistency standards by asking every single asthma patient about possible triggers for her asthma and by educating every single asthma patient about appropriate responses to early asthma symptoms, the results may not meet the Six Sigma standard of fewer than three asthma patients per million with complications, but we know they can lead to a 70 to 80 percent reduction in asthma crisis. Six Sigma–like provider performance for asthma care can have huge positive impacts on patient status and patient outcomes.

Buyer-Driven Improvements

To achieve those kinds of highly positive results, we need the kind of systems-based care that prevents significant care linkage deficiencies. Some health plans and organized care systems (including Kaiser Permanente) undertake extensive and systematic asthma intervention programs as a matter of course. But many unlinked providers do not use or have access to that kind of systematic approach, and patients suffer as a result.

What can be done where there is no care system of any kind currently taking accountability for reducing the number of asthma attacks? Chapter Six discusses a market model where a responsible entity working from either electronic medical records or the claims payment system electronic personal health record aggregated database can see and influence which providers are providing complete care. There is an obvious need for such a responsible entity to work to ensure that there are direct follow-up communications to asthma patients with frequent asthma problems.

Who will make sure that kind of linked care is implemented? In Chapter Seven, I discuss the role of buyers. I believe that the role of the buyer will be essential to true health care reform.

Successful asthma crisis interventions are far more likely to happen if the primary purchasers of care—the employers and government agencies who purchase benefits—insist on the existence of some functional level of fully linked, medically appropriate precrisis care as a condition of doing business with whatever health plans or benefit administrators that they use to run their benefits programs. Why is buyer intervention necessary? Because most independent care providers left to their own devices will not somehow magically migrate to strategically integrated care or to any form of team-based care delivery on their own. The history and current status of American health care has already proven that to be true. And it's not hard to see why. I made this point earlier, but let me make it one more time.

There are no current financial rewards paid or given to independent caregivers for that kind of provider integration, and there are some actual financial barriers to fully integrated best care for asthma patients. Again, run the numbers and look at the contrasts. Patients might pay a doctor $100 for an asthma prevention visit and another $200 for their inhaler prescription. An ER visit, on the other hand, can generate $2,000 to $4,000 in provider revenue and a full-boat hospitalization could generate from $10,000 to $40,000 in caregiver revenue. If money incents behavior, where are we as a society putting our money today? It's not in preventing asthma attacks—even though America is in an asthma epidemic.

Those financial rewards need to be reengineered by each payer and carrier so that responsible entities are putting in place a workable path to an appropriate level of integrated care for asthma patients.

Internet-Driven Care

The other likely and workable leverage point we need to use far more often and effectively to improve asthma care is the development of good information that is made available directly to asthma patients through the Internet. The Internet can be our best friend in getting key information about asthma and other chronic diseases to individual patients. Everybody wants to know how to use best care for their own health problem. People will do the right thing fairly consistently when they know clearly what the right thing to do is.

Good and credible health care web sites, such as the one in Box 4.1, can explain appropriate asthma care approaches directly to the patients, giving the patients information that can be used to encourage appropriate patient behavior and to trigger clear communication with their doctors about possible treatment approaches. Rather than resist or resent the use of the Internet as a source of information for patients about care, the best caregivers should direct their patients to the best web sites. The very best caregivers and health plans should, will, and do use websites as a patient education tool. We need to get even better at that whole strategy if we really expect to improve the outcomes of care.

Especially as high-speed Internet becomes widely available, patients with significant diagnoses increasingly tend to go to the Internet to learn more about their disease. We need as a nation to

Box 4.1. Asthma Information and Virtual Consultation.

The American Lung Association is a great place to start looking for patient information, at www.lungusa.org. The American Lung Association also offers a virtual consultation service called the NexProfiler Treatment Option Tool. It's available at http://www.lungusa.org/site/pp.asp?c_dvLUK9O0E&b=38472.

take advantage of that tendency to use the web to be sure that patients receive valid, credible, and useful information that can help each individual be a better and more discerning value-based customer with his care provider.

The web is still a very underutilized tool when it comes to direct patient care. That will change. Ideally, as new levels of individual patient care information become electronically available to patients, employers and plan administrators should deliberately, carefully, and effectively facilitate patient access to specific, very useful web tools.

Ideally, those tools will use the patient's newly electronic personal health information in the context of various expert algorithms that will give patients access to a "virtual consult" about their disease. These interactive web sites will help patients get a second opinion about their care. I predict and expect that the electronic second opinion process will become an industry unto itself, with well-informed patients being one result.

Early versions of those virtual consult tools exist now. Some are good and some are weak. The good ones need to be reinforced, and access to them should be facilitated so that the patients who do not have the benefit of a live, face-to-face multispecialty care team can have the computer equivalent of a *Consumer Reports* database for discussing and resolving key care disease issues with their physician.

Asthma is a condition that particularly lends itself to that electronic support kit. Protocols exist. Best care expectations can be set. Prescription options are known. Deviations from best care can be detected and dealt with, both by patients and by computer database monitoring mechanisms. Patients can and should be appropriately involved in the entire process.

Asthma's Bottom Line

We should be able to improve the health of people with asthma and cut the overall cost of asthma care if we proceed strategically to create team-based general care, educate all people with asthma on the most effective self-help for their disease, support written care plans, and then reward care administrators for improving compliance with asthma care best practices.

There are huge opportunities for care improvement, not just for individuals but for communities. The PHR databases will give us a whole new opportunity to look at asthma care and case loads by zip code, comorbidity, age, weight, and dozens of other correlations of fact and demographics. Community health agendas can have real impact. The research potential is golden. If we could run the PHR database for an entire community to discover that the highest rate of asthma cases sorted by zip code happens most often to the people who live closest to the center of town or closest to the river, there could be something to learn from that data that could help improve care for everyone. And that data could let communities target their asthma prevention and treatment resources to the sites and caregivers with the greatest potential benefit.

It's entirely possible that in the future entire communities could take on asthma as a community health agenda, targeting significant reductions in the asthma burden placed on identified populations, neighborhoods, and age groups. Those kinds of campaigns would be facilitated by access to communitywide data about asthma care and by a history of success in using good treatment tools to prevent crisis and improve care.

Diabetes

Asthma is a major problem in America. Diabetes is an even bigger problem.

Diabetes is the single most important chronic condition in America today relative to both patient health and the cost of care because of its explosive growth over the past quarter century. It affects the most people and, with its comorbidities, costs the most money. In 1980, 6 million Americans had diabetes. Today, almost 21 million do—and that number is growing by more than a million every year.[20]

As I noted earlier, diabetes is now the number-one cause of kidney failure. Each year, between 12,000 and 24,000 adults go blind from diabetic retinal disease, and at least 80,000 people have a lower limb amputation as a result of diabetes.[21] It's the number-one comorbidity associated with death from heart disease, and the risk of stroke is two to four times higher for people with diabetes.[22] New evidence points to the possibility that diabetes also increases the risk of developing Alzheimer's disease.[23]

The total direct and indirect costs of diabetes in the United States are $132 billion.[24] People with diabetes alone spend more than 32 percent of all the monies spent on patients by Medicare.[25]

And yet the most recent RAND study showed that patients with diabetes receive only 45 percent of recommended care.[26] That's both a terrible indictment of the inconsistencies of the current American health care delivery nonsystem and an excellent opportunity for change. If those same studies had shown that almost all people with diabetes in America today already received best, optimal, efficient, and completely appropriate care, the opportunity for real improvement in care outcomes and cost would obviously be pretty modest. But when people with diabetes incur all of those costs and experience all of those debilitating complications yet care is measurably inadequate and incomplete for the majority of them, then it would be immoral, irresponsible, and illogical not to explore significant opportunities for systematic improvement.

Preventing Diabetes

Before talking about those opportunities, let's discuss why diabetes is growing so rapidly. The answer? Personal health choices. Americans are increasingly obese and inert. Figures 4.2, 4.3, and 4.4 make this point graphically. Over sixty million people—more than 30 percent of the adult population—are obese,[27] and almost 90 percent of people with Type 2 diabetes are overweight.[28] Diabetes is a disease that is very often triggered by people being overweight and inactive. Those are not the only causes of diabetes—many of the people who

Figure 4.2. Prevalence of Obesity in the United States, 1985.

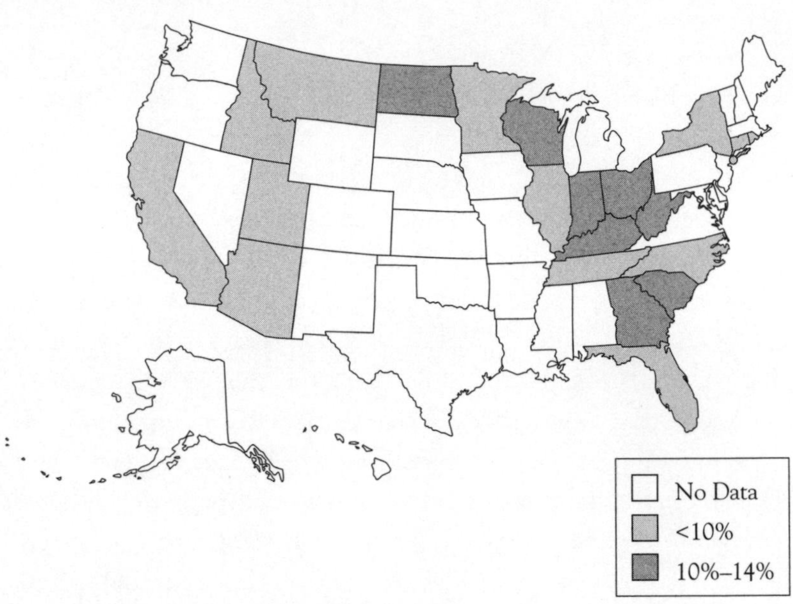

Source: Division of Nutrition and Physical Activity, National Center for Chronic Disease Prevention and Health Promotion, "Overweight and Obesity: Obesity Trends—U. S. Obesity Trends 1985-2005." Bethesda, Md.: Centers for Disease Control, 2006.

develop diabetes are both slender and active—but good studies show that if Americans were 5 to 10 percent thinner and simply walked as little as thirty minutes a day, the incidence of Type 2 diabetes in this country could be cut by more than half.[29]

Some people believe the reduction could be even greater. A famous study done of Pima Indians on the Mexican-American border studied people from the same tribe, with the same genetic makeup, who had very different lifestyles and very different diets, depending on whether they lived on the Mexican or American side of the border. By age sixty-five, more than half of the American Pima Indians had diabetes. By that same age, less than 10 percent

Figure 4.3. Prevalence of Obesity in the United States, 1995.

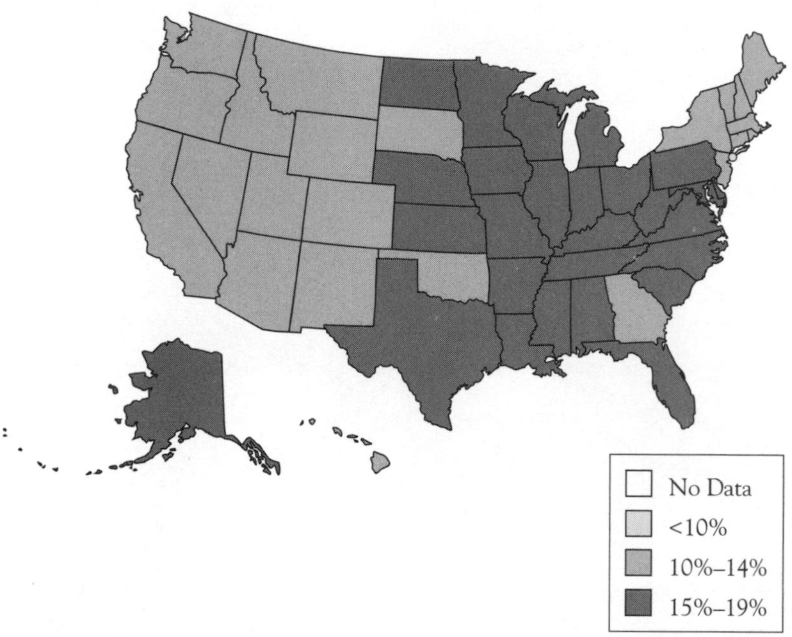

Source: Division of Nutrition and Physical Activity, National Center for Chronic Disease Prevention and Health Promotion, "Overweight and Obesity: Obesity Trends—U. S. Obesity Trends 1985-2005." Bethesda, Md.: Centers for Disease Control, 2006.

of the Mexican Pima Indians had diabetes. The difference in disease burden was attributable to diet and activity levels—not genetics.[30] One tribe. One gene pool. Two diets. Two levels of activity. Two very different results. There was no fast food on the Mexican side of the border.

Research showing the links between people with diabetes, diet, weight, and activity levels can be found on the web. The Diabetes Prevention Program study followed 3,200 people who were overweight and had impaired glucose tolerance—both well-known risk factors for developing diabetes.[31] For three years, subjects were placed in three groups. Group 1 received intensive training in diet,

Figure 4.4. Prevalence of Obesity in the United States, 2005.

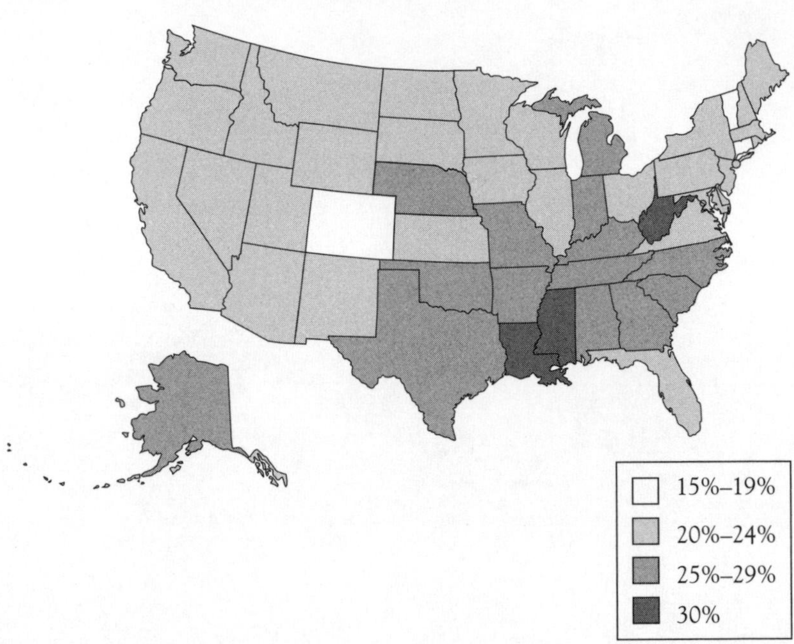

Source: Division of Nutrition and Physical Activity, National Center for Chronic Disease Prevention and Health Promotion, "Overweight and Obesity: Obesity Trends—U. S. Obesity Trends 1985-2005." Bethesda, Md.: Centers for Disease Control, 2006.

exercise, and behavior modification. They ate less fat and fewer calories and exercised for 150 minutes a week, aiming to lose 7 percent of their body weight. Group 2 received metformin, an oral diabetes drug. Group 3 received a placebo.

The results were stunning. The people in Group 1 reduced their risk of developing diabetes by 58 percent. People over the age of 60 did even better, reducing their risk by 71 percent. Group 2 participants reduced their risk by only 31 percent. Diet and exercise work to prevent diabetes.

The American Diabetes Association has great information on diabetes research.[32] We know how to prevent diabetes. The information is out there and available. Health care needs to take advantage of it.

Changing Care Culture

The very best long-term strategy for American health care should be to encourage and facilitate lifestyle changes for people who are at risk of diabetes in order to decrease the possibility that they will develop diabetes. That kind of approach takes a consistent, effective, individually targeted, systematic communications effort. Most health care providers aren't organized systematically, so they can't provide this kind of systematic care. To achieve that level of care will take a cultural change effort, not just a care delivery change effort. But the care system can help create that cultural change.

Studies show that patients are influenced by what they hear directly from their caregivers.[33] We need highly credible doctors, nurses, and health educators talking to patients in targeted and effective ways to help people make the lifestyle changes necessary to avoid diabetes. We also need community leaders who are willing to take on lifestyle issues like obesity and inactivity as a public health agenda—a real opportunity to make lives better for a great many people.

We are beginning to see some real leadership in those areas. America on the Move is a national nonprofit organization that seeks to improve the health and quality of life for Americans by promoting healthful eating and active living.[34] The state of Colorado has been on board since 2001, and they have already seen the results: they were one of only four states with a prevalence of obesity less than 20 percent in 2005.[35] Shape Up America! is another nonprofit organization founded by C. Everett Koop in 1994 dedicated to raising awareness of obesity as a health issue and to providing responsible information on healthy weight management. Shape Up America! promotes the ten thousand steps a day approach to becoming more active.[36]

We need that kind of community-based leadership to continue. We need campaigns to do things as basic as removing soda pop from school cafeterias and reintroducing physical education classes for students. Workplace exercise programs should be encouraged as well.

Diabetes Care Requires a Team Effort

Prevention is our best longer-term strategy for reducing the complications and expense of diabetes. On the more immediate horizon, we need to do a much better job helping people who already have diabetes to avoid the complications of that disease.

While no two people with diabetes will be the same, treatment of diabetes generally includes controlling blood sugar levels through a combination of diet, weight loss, exercise, and, as needed, medications. Other associated health issues such as blood pressure control and cholesterol control must also be addressed. Patients with diabetes need regular monitoring of their blood sugar, weight, cholesterol, and kidney function. They also need intermittent visits with their main diabetes doctor, whether a primary care or specialty physician, to monitor their progress and check for other potential problems such as nerve damage and skin breakdown. People with diabetes also need to see an eye doctor regularly to check for any diabetes-caused eye damage. While diabetes can damage many organs and tissues, close attention to treatment and periodic monitoring can detect changes early and allow a better chance of avoiding serious complications.

In order to achieve that level of medical support for people with diabetes, we need effective, consistent, and dependable systems to remind the caregivers and patients what tests need to be done and what follow-up care is needed when the tests show problematic results. Best care for diabetes takes a coordinated team of dedicated people—doctors, dieticians, health educators, the patient, and her family—along with good communication and computer systems to help coordinate and track appropriate care.

Americans with diabetes suffer constantly from care linkage deficiencies. Caregivers forget to order tests. Patients with comorbidities generally receive little or no direct support for their diabetic care from the caregivers treating their other diseases. Too many cardiologists, for example, don't interact with or ensure follow-up for tests the patient may need for foot care, eye care, or blood sugar control. Major opportunities for care improvement and care coordination are missed. Often.

This is another area where each patient should be encouraged and educated by Internet support systems to get all key tests and checkups done, and to hold their caregiver or caregivers accountable for delivering systematic, protocol-driven care. Informed patients can help reform the system and create a consistency of care that has a powerful spill-over impact on their own health and their caregivers' process of care.

The potential cost savings for diabetes is huge. The cumulative impact of best care practices is huge all by itself. A third of kidney failure patients with diabetes would not have lost their kidneys with appropriate care and prior behavior changes.[37] Foot care programs that include regular examinations and patient education could prevent up to 85 percent of diabetes-related amputations.[38] Regular eye exams and timely treatment could prevent up to 90 percent of diabetes-related blindness.[39] In other words, the complications of diabetes can be cut by 33 percent to 90 percent using systematic best care. Patients who do as little as walk thirty minutes or so a day while watching their fat and calorie intake can reduce the incidence of Type 2 diabetes by nearly half. The opportunities are immense, and the price we pay for not handling diabetes effectively is huge. Diabetes is, in the words of my personal cardiologist, "The mother of all diseases—the comorbidity that ties together the other main diseases and makes them all a lot worse."

We can do better—and with systematic approaches, we will do better.

Coronary Artery Disease

Coronary artery disease is the other major chronic disease that we need to deal with far more effectively and consistently as a country. Coronary artery disease is the single largest killer of American men and women. Nearly every minute, an American man or woman dies from coronary heart disease.[40]

We already discussed congestive heart failure. Coronary artery disease is not the same as congestive heart failure. In congestive heart failure, the heart muscle grows weak and eventually fails. In coronary artery disease, the problem is not with the heart muscle itself, but with the arteries that lead to the heart. When they become clogged, blood cannot get to the heart and the heart muscle dies from lack of oxygen. The degree of clogging of American arteries is amazing, again fueled by our diet and our sad lack of physical activity. Every year, an estimated 700,000 Americans have a first heart attack, and 500,000 have a subsequent attack.[41] The direct and indirect costs of heart disease are estimated at $142.5 billion a year.[42] As a nation, we spend more than a quarter of a million dollars *every minute* on heart disease.

Preventing Heart Attacks

Even more than diabetes, coronary artery disease should be a preventable medical condition. Nine risk factors account for 90 percent of the risk of an initial heart attack: cigarette smoking, high blood cholesterol levels, hypertension, diabetes, obesity, a lack of physical activity, low intake of fruits and vegetables, alcohol overconsumption, and psychosocial factors.[43] Most people who develop the disease would not have gotten it if their diets had been better and their activity levels higher.

Good health habits are the best defense against heart disease. What's exciting, however, is that coronary artery disease can be prevented or delayed using prescription drugs. There is a vast body of evidence that tells us that we can prevent heart attacks for many people if we use blood pressure medications, cholesterol-lowering drugs, and aspirin.[44] The responses can be relatively quick.

One of our Kaiser Permanente projects simply added three drugs to the daily intake of thousands of heart patients. Those three drugs were aspirin, lovastatin (a cholesterol-lowering drug), and lisinopril (a blood pressure medication). Based on modeling through our Kaiser Permanente Archimedes System and early results, we expect the number of heart attacks to drop by over half among people at risk.[45]

A Personal Story

I can speak about this particular disease from some very personal experience. I have had very high cholesterol for years that I was recently trying to bring under control with some medication. That was the only good news. I've been in my current job for roughly four years. Over that time frame, due to bad scheduling, a lot of travel, and a personal unwillingness to force myself to find time to exercise, I gained fifty pounds and had a life almost devoid of physical activity. I haven't been on either of my sail boards in four years, and my kayak in California hasn't left my garage in three years. I have time to write this book right now because I am in the final stages of recovery therapy after a heart attack followed by a quadruple coronary artery bypass. I had a couple of heart arteries clogged at roughly 90 percent and a fourth at 99 percent. They tell me that 90 percent clogged isn't good.

One of the great things about working in the San Francisco Bay Area is the superb set of local restaurants and cooks. Unfortunately, as wonderful as the local cheese carts may be from a taste perspective, they aren't entirely heart healthy. So I have now gotten religious on the issue of healthy living at a very personal level. I've given up red meat for at least a year. I'm eating food that Dean Ornish would recommend. I'm on a couple of medications. My total cholesterol is now barely over 100. I am exercising five to seven days a week, and working to get my newly replumbed heart strong enough for just about any eventuality.

I was lucky. My heart damage could have been far worse. The surgery seems to have been a complete success. With that new plumbing, I hope to have quite a few useful years. But I definitely have personally become part of the 1 percent of our population who utilized 35 percent of the care dollars this year. What I need to do now is adhere rigorously to all the personal accountability healthy behavior steps necessary to make sure that I don't rejoin the top 1 percent anytime soon.

My story shows that we can improve, personally and systemically. If I do everything the right way now and keep doing it, I should be in maintenance mode for many years to come. If I went back to my old bad weight, picked up my old diet, and stopped my current medications, the likelihood of me having a second heart attack very soon would be several times higher.

That's the challenge and the opportunity.

Continuously Improving Quality

In one of our Kaiser Permanente regions, we started a systematic computer-supported process of making sure that every heart patient got every piece of appropriate medication, counsel, and care according to best practices. It was a Six Sigma–like pilot study, with the goal of having 100 percent of the diagnosed heart patients getting the right attention at every single visit from the caregivers. Computers supported the process by reminding the caregivers what needed to be done for each patient at each visit. One hundred percent caregiver consistency is obviously not enough to ensure 100 percent patient success or best care compliance, because patients make their own decisions, but the actual success levels for the pilot were amazing. Over three years, the death rate from heart disease for our patients in that pilot region dropped to 30 percent less than the state average.[46]

Health care can be improved. The challenge is to do it consistently and systematically, not incidentally and haphazardly. Continuous quality improvement approaches are needed. Consistent best practices are the key. Using the computer to remind the doctors and nurses what tests were needed and whether prescriptions were being filled was the breakthrough tool for that pilot program.

Without a computerized reminder system, complete caregiver consistency is impossible, and results at this level are unattainable.

Coronary artery disease can be prevented, and it can be treated in ways that slow the progression of the disease and mitigate the symptoms. However, that kind of care has to be done systematically or it won't be done effectively. As a society and as a health care marketplace we need to track whether or not care is being delivered appropriately, and we need to offer reminders to patients and caregivers about the best treatments and optimal behaviors.

Simply letting heart attacks happen and then responding to the crises is not the right strategy for American health care. That's how this country got to the position we are in now—the most expensive care delivery infrastructure in the world.

Depression

The fifth chronic disease that creates real cost and quality of life problems is depression. By the year 2020, depression is expected to be second only to heart disease as a source of the overall mortality and disability burden of disease around the world.[47] More than fifteen million Americans have depression, making it the fourth most prevalent chronic condition.[48] Depression is intimately related to other chronic diseases and complicates their care, often leading to poorer outcomes and more expensive treatment. Only one in four people have depression alone; on average, a person with depression has three other chronic conditions.[49]

Nearly 50 percent of asthma patients may also suffer from depression.[50] Depression is twice as prevalent among people with diabetes as it is in the general population.[51] The relationship between depression and heart disease begs the question of whether the chicken or the egg came first. People with depression have an approximately 60 percent greater risk of developing heart disease than do people without depression,[52] and people with a history of depression are more than four times more likely to have a heart attack than those with no history of depression.[53] Roughly one in three people who've had a heart attack also suffer from major depression, which reduces the likelihood that they'll adhere to recommended lifestyle and behavioral changes.[54]

It probably shouldn't be a surprise that many of our highest-cost patients have depression as either a solo diagnosis or as a comorbidity. The estimated direct costs of depression are $77 billion.[55] The estimated overall cost of depression to U.S. employers is staggering. The cost of lost productive work time is very conservatively estimated at $44 billion,[56] and the costs of health care for depressed employees are nearly twice those of workers who are not depressed.[57] Counting lost time from the job, depression can cost many billions of dollars.

So what can be done to alleviate the problem? Again, a systematic approach is the key. Early and accurate diagnosis is an extremely important first step. Depression obviously can't be dealt with until it's on the table for both the caregiver and the patient. Once diagnosed, both talk therapy and various prescription treatments can be extremely useful.

A major key to patient improvement when prescriptions are the treatment of choice is systematic follow-up to make sure the prescriptions are being filled and used. Because 30 percent of patients suffering from depression don't start or drop out of medication treatment,[58] the best approach for better health outcomes is a feedback loop to let the caregiver know whether or not prescriptions are being filled. If they are not being filled, then that's an issue that needs to be dealt with between the caregiver and the patient. Again, provider consistency, care system follow up, and patient focus are the key performance metrics.

This is another instance where the computer can help. Both electronic medical records and personal health record systems can be useful for tracking whether or not prescriptions were actually filled or renewed. Research projects in those areas of performance need to be done.

The care of people with depression will, I believe, evolve into an even more effective model as the health care infrastructure evolves into more systematic approaches to all major diseases. Depression isn't leading that effort, but I expect that it will benefit as well from systematic thought processes and care reinforcement.

Consistent Follow-Up Is Key

Those are the big five chronic conditions that drive health care costs. Simple, consistent, science-based follow-up in each area has the potential for huge savings. A mere 10 percent savings for just 0.5 percent of American patients would reduce the health care bill for America by many billions of dollars—more than enough to fund total and universal health care coverage for the uninsured.

A key fact to remember in dealing with each of those conditions is that optimal results will come from patients working with their doctors and care teams, having appropriate tests done, filling their prescriptions, and reliably taking their medication. Consistent and dependable follow-up care is key, and that follow-up care is most likely to happen in a consistent way if it is supported by a computer system set up to facilitate and support consistent care. That computer system can be the electronic medical record (EMR) of a vertically integrated care system like Kaiser Permanente, or it can be driven from the amalgamated personal health record (PHR) database compiled from claims payment data by various insurance companies and self-insurance employers. The EMR data is more complete, but, as discussed in the last chapter, the PHR data is far better than nothing and should be used as soon as that database becomes available.

If we did nothing other than focus effectively on the opportunities presented by chronic care for the next several years, we would be making huge progress in both improving care and reducing the overall costs of care in this country.

What About Acute Conditions?

Most of America's health care costs come from chronic diseases. That doesn't mean, however, that acute conditions don't cost money. The most expensive acute care conditions in total make up roughly 30 percent of American health care spending.[59] They also present care delivery improvement opportunities.

The most expensive acute care conditions are cancer care, maternity and childbirth-related care, and trauma care.[60] A more systematic, market-facing, value-based care delivery system could make significant progress in both cost containment and quality improvement in each of those areas.

Maternity Care

Childbirth is a good example. In maternity care, huge expenses occur from a relatively small number of preterm births, roughly 12 percent of all deliveries.[61] Some of those cases can, all by themselves, cost upwards of a million dollars. Yet our infant mortality levels in this country are not particularly good in comparison to other countries. We rank thirty-fifth in infant mortality in the world.[62]

What can we do to improve those numbers? We can do a much better job of systematically and consistently identifying which mothers are at highest risk for having a preterm baby, and we can then work closely with each high-risk mother to significantly reduce her risk. Half of those preterm births could be avoided by effectively identifying high-risk mothers and then putting forth an equally effective effort to help each high-risk mother reduce her risk factors and be personally prepared for quick and systematic intervention if the baby starts to come early.[63]

Medical techniques can stop some preterm labor and keep many premature births from happening. That's important, because full-term babies tend to be much healthier. Babies born very prematurely are not only at risk of death, they are also often very much at risk of lifelong health problems that can make their lives unpleasant and hard. For instance, roughly 10 percent of premature babies experience intraventricular hemorrhage—or bleeding into the brain—which can result in brain damage.[64]

Having a healthy full-term baby is a goal to be sought after. However, available labor-delay techniques will be effective only if each expectant mother knows exactly what the signs of preterm labor are and exactly what to do about them if they should occur.

Better prenatal care is key to the process. First, we must make sure that care is available to all women. That often requires insurance coverage for expectant mothers so that prenatal care is available and affordable. Uninsured women tend not to receive needed prenatal care. More on that point in Chapter Eleven of this book.

In the longer term, we need a systematic plan aimed at using our entire new tool kit to help reduce the number of preterm births. Again, the application of Six Sigma–like thought processes to the entire pregnancy process yields quick and logical conclusions about the opportunity for high-leverage, high-value interventions. It will take the kind of system outlined in Chapter Six to fully implement those processes.

Cancer

Cancer is another important area where care improvements could be derived in part from market forces. There is too much inconsistency in cancer care. The RAND studies showed that breast cancer patients received 86 percent of recommended care.[65] The good news is that 86 percent was the highest performance score for any area of American health care that was reviewed. The bad news is that study tells us that recommended care is not delivered 14 percent of the time. Even worse, patients with colorectal cancer received only 54 percent of recommended care.

There's no reason to believe that there are not comparable or greater variations in care approaches for the other two cancers that have the largest volume and cost—prostate cancer and lung cancer—even though they weren't studied. Minimally, consumers ought to have access to the best available information about current care alternatives and best practices for the treatment of each cancer. Consumers also should have scorecards showing, for example, the comparative life expectancy success rate for Stage III lung cancer patients among local oncologists. Differences exist. Not all caregivers end up with the same success rate for the treatment.

Box 4.2 demonstrates how different caregiver success and survival rates can be for the inherited disease cystic fibrosis. The same difference in success rates can occur in cancer treatment as well. We know that the five-year difference in breast cancer mortality can vary by up to 60 percent depending on which hospitals and surgery teams did the breast surgery.[66] Some people might find a 60 percent difference in five year mortality rates to be meaningful data. We should want that level of data available to patients and caregivers in our health care marketplace at multiple levels. It will take a couple of years to get that level of data ready, but it is a doable goal if we put in place an electronic health record system or even an aggregated claims-based PHR database. With that kind of standardized aggregated database we should be able to show relatively soon that if you have your lung cancer treated by Dr. Smith, you will live, on average four months, where, if you have lung cancer treated by Dr. Jones, you will live, on average, eight months. Lung cancer is a disease where relative survival rate information can be hugely important to people making what are very often the last major decisions in their lives. Knowing the relative survival time frames both for specific treatments and specific caregivers can be immeasurably valuable information.

Box 4.2. Varying Outcomes for Cystic Fibrosis.

Cystic fibrosis is a life-threatening disease that causes severe lung damage and nutritional deficiencies. An inherited condition, cystic fibrosis affects cells that produce mucus, sweat, saliva, and dietary juices. It cannot be cured, and respiratory failure is a deadly complication of cystic fibrosis. The Cystic Fibrosis Foundation keeps track of long-term survival rates from all 117 certified cystic fibrosis treatment care centers. All are rigorously certified and involve highly expert caregivers. But the life expectancy at the highest-performing center is 47 years, 14 years longer than the median life expectancy of 33 for all 117 centers.

Source: A. Gawande, "The Bell Curve," *New Yorker*, Dec. 6, 2004.

Is measuring performance really where we should place our priorities relative to tracking and improving care? Let me take that question to a very personal level. If you were personally diagnosed today with lung cancer, would you want to know that kind of relative and comparative survival rate information? Of course you would. The caregivers themselves would also find it very useful to know that another doctor down the street kept their lung cancer patients alive three times longer. Every single doctor wants to deliver best care. A great learning would occur among physicians once valid comparative data became available. Market forces would very directly impact care if that happened. But only if the right data is made available, so true value-based purchasing decisions can be made by patients. Market forces will not impact lung cancer treatment programs—or any other cancer treatment approaches—until that comparative data exists.

I want to stress that variations in care outcomes do not exist because any oncologists anywhere are trying to deliver inappropriate or less effective care. None are. Every oncologist believes he or she is delivering the best care to his or her patients—but without data, the oncologists have no way of knowing if their belief is correct. Remember in Chapter Two we saw that radiologists who read mammograms could not and did not improve their personal success rate at reading mammograms until it became known that other radiologists were doing a measurably better job. Until that fact was known, every single radiologist assumed and believed completely that his or her personal performance was in fact as good as that particular job could be done. Right now, I am sure that every oncologist in America believes he or she is doing the best job and getting the best results. The amount of credible data available to help each oncologist know whether or not that is actually true should be expanded, like the database for the mammogram-reading radiologists.

On a broader scale, if consumers could check to see which oncologists help create the longest life expectancy for Stage III lung cancer patients, that would only be one piece of valuable information that needs to be considered in making important care decisions. Ideally, that same database should measure patient satisfaction with each oncologist, and the market model should facilitate communication from the caregivers about their personal approach to care. In an optimal setting, it should be clear from both the doctor's own words and patient testimonials how the doctor deals with delicate but extremely important issues like using multiple, painful treatments that are statistically unlikely to succeed for end-of-life care.

Some cancer treatments have wonderful success rates. Others are used in terminal patients with a very low likelihood of success. Those facts need to be understood. In some cases, the doctors define the success of a given treatment or surgery not by whether or not it cures anything, but by whether it has some estimated chance of adding days or weeks or even months to a person's life span. Sometimes those specific surgery treatments that might add weeks of life can be painful debilitators and create mandatory patient isolation. And then the final result is exactly the same. The patient dies. What is the value to each patient of those additional survival times? Shouldn't the patient clearly know the trade-off between intense debilitation and additional weeks of life? Shouldn't we be measuring exactly how long the average lung cancer surgery patient lives compared to the chemo patient, the radiation patient, the full-boat patient, and the patient who chooses no care at all other than pain relief? Those measurements need to be done. Patients need to know the results. Buyers should insist that the health care products they purchase will develop and provide that kind of data.

Those types of facts and issues all should be far better known by patients than they are now. If you personally had a terminal cancer, wouldn't you like to know how the doctor you are choosing deals with those issues? And wouldn't you like to know what the real survival extension numbers are for your disease? A doctor with a slightly shorter survival period for their average Stage III cancer patients, but a much higher use of hospice care, pain controls, and a very respectful approach to end-of-life issues could be a choice we might individually like to make. Or we might choose a more heroic but low-probability, radical treatment approach that possibly extends life by some hopefully longer period of time.

As patients, we need to be able to make timely, informed choices. It's our life. Our personal cancer care approach can be the last set of real choices we get to make. We should, I believe, be able to make them in the most informed way. If we want a doctor who will do every last surgery because one might work, we should be able to make that choice. If we want a doctor who will tell us when the situation is hopeless and it's time to make a graceful exit, then we should be able to make that choice as well. The choice should be ours—and we should have enough information to make that choice well.

The health care marketplace for cancer care should be data-rich and patient-focused.

Cancer and maternity care are just two of an array of acute health care conditions where we could and should create far better performance measures for our caregivers and far better information flows for our patients as part of a new health care reform agenda. If we decide to use the aggregated personal health record data set from each community to measure the relative success of caregivers who use each approach, we could manage to accelerate the process of creating market-based health care buying significantly. It will take a few years to get that full database in place, so we need to start now, designing the specific questions we want that database to answer.

Patient Financial Incentives: Deductibles and Chronic Care

One last thought on the topic of needed care for the five chronic diseases that consume the bulk of our health care dollar. A number of economists have theorized that patients will make better and often less expensive choices about their health care usage if each patient has financial "skin in the game"—a personal economic incentive to spend money more frugally.[67] The usual financial incentive that is being proposed today by some health care economists, some health insurance companies, and a few political leaders to accomplish that particular economic incentive goal is to give people a high-deductible benefit plan, where the patient must pay out of his or her own pocket for the first thousand, two thousand, or three thousand dollars worth of personal care.[68]

High-Deductible Plans

The theory is that most current health insurance benefit packages are very rich, and that people are therefore so insulated from any direct care costs by their health insurance benefits that care is, for all practical purposes, free to the consumer. Those economists argue that people tend not to value a "free" good. They also argue—I think accurately—that when patients are totally insulated from the costs of care, then patients are much less likely to price shop and much less likely to pick a less expensive care alternative. People will, they say, price shop when people have to directly pay the relevant prices for care out of their own pocket. That is, I believe, true.

The cost difference between a clinic that charges $80.00 for a primary care visit and another clinic that charges $120.00 for that same office visit might cause patients who are paying directly out of pocket for their care to select the less expensive $80.00 provider. However, when insurance pays in full for both visits and the patient pays only a $15.00 copay for either visit, then the insurance coverage completely eliminates the cost difference between the two providers and the patient has no financial reason to select the better-priced caregiver. In fact, if the patient who will pay only the $15.00 copay happens to learn that one doctor charges $120.00 for an office visit and the other charges $80.00, the patient may chose the $120.00 physician on the generic theory that higher-cost care must also be higher-quality care and therefore it is better and smarter to pay the same flat copay and get care from the more expensive provider.

So obviously using a flat copayment as an insurance benefit does not encourage the selection of lower-cost office visits. A cost-sharing mechanism is needed to achieve that goal. One current school of thought is that the way to introduce cost-based decision making into health care might be by eliminating flat copayments and instead introducing significant front-end deductibles to the health care benefit package for employees. With the new deductible plans, the patients must pay the first thousand or so dollars of care out of their own pocket. New laws set up to encourage that particular type of benefit package allow patients to place part of their paycheck into a special medical savings account (called the health savings account), with the ability to use that set-aside money to pay the deductible amounts when care is actually needed and purchased.[69] The relevant theory behind that benefit design is that patients will pay more attention to cost differences when those costs are paid directly and totally by the patient.

The cost-sharing theory is right as a theory. Patients will often choose the cheaper option. But what is cheaper in health care is not always obvious. As we have seen, sometimes it is cheaper to spend money up front on prevention than at the back end when a patient is in crisis.

Unexpected Outcomes: Hospital Choices

The key question to ask is about these high-deductible plans is, What are the overall consequences of the consumer-based decisions they provoke? Do patients make smart choices as a result of that out-of-pocket expense? The decisions made by patients in these circumstances create both good news and bad news.

Interestingly, for some types of health care decisions, a $1,000 or even $2,000 deductible can create a set of perverse economic issues very similar to the ones created by flat copayments for clinical office visits. Hospital costs are a major health care cost factor, for example. How does a deductible benefit package influence consumers in their choice of hospitals?

When one hospital costs $5,000 a day for care and the hospital across the street performs the same services for $10,000 a day, even a $3,000 dollar deductible becomes economically irrelevant instantly for either hospital choice if the patient will need to stay for a full day. Do the math. The $3,000 deductible is spent in the first fifteen hours in Hospital #1, and it is spent in the first seven hours in Hospital #2. In either hospital, for all practical purposes, the full deductible is used up immediately. It's a completely sunk cost for the patient on day one in either hospital. So both hospitals actually cost a flat $3,000 to the patient—no personal cost difference at all. The patient obviously has no incentive to select a lower-cost hospital based on the deductible. In fact, it may be the reverse. Some consumers are likely to say, "If I have to spend the first $3,000 myself, do I want to use my fixed amount of money to buy a $5,000 hospital day or a $10,000 hospital day?"

If it were a hotel purchase, what would you do? "Here's the new expense account deal," your employer says. "You need to pay the first $300 yourself each night as a hotel room deductible. You decide whether you want to stay in a $500 a night hotel room or a $1,000 per night hotel room. You pick. Then you pay a flat $300 for either room. I'll pay the difference."

People might well tend to believe that a $1,000 a night room could be nicer in some ways than a $500 room, so some employees in those circumstances might pick the more expensive room. Just because it's more expensive. Hospital choices made using the fixed deductible benefit model are subject to a similar thought process. There are similar price issues for decisions like choice of surgeon or even which MRI to use. Deductibles only work if the unit of care being purchased costs less than the deductible. Once all of the relevant care alternatives for the patient cost more than the patient's deductible, the value of the deductible to sway decision making diminishes. A pure deductible therefore often does not directly encourage or incent wise price shopping when it comes to really big-ticket health care items.

Unexpected Outcomes: Preventive and Maintenance Care

Deductibles do, however, influence many choices on smaller-ticket items. If the deductible exceeds the cost of the service being considered, then the price of the service is very relevant to the patient.

Again, as noted earlier, that also can be either good news or bad news. Think again about who spends the vast majority of our health care dollars. Those dollars are spent mostly by people with chronic diseases. Remember how many drugs are used to prevent or delay the most expensive crisis stages of chronic diseases. When we need people to buy and use a medication to prevent asthma attacks, to avoid second heart attacks, or to ward off an expensive, life-threatening congestive heart failure crisis, then we want people to have an incentive to fill those prescriptions. Creating a direct financial barrier to the purchase of those provably effective prescriptions might not be the smartest thing to do either economically or medically. Economic incentives do influence decisions. The underlying economic theory is entirely valid that out-of-pocket expense levels directly influence patient decisions about health care purchases. Evidence shows, in fact, that chronic care patients faced with new insurance benefit deductibles often do exactly what the deductibles were set up to encourage them to do—they avoid making purchases. Unfortunately, many of the chronic care patients then make cost-based decisions not to buy their needed chronic care treatment drugs. Those same patients too often also decide not to get a full set of follow-up exams, and they decide not to run and pay for basic tests needed to monitor their condition. Those are not decisions we really want chronic care patients to make.

That isn't a theoretical conclusion. We did a significant study at Kaiser Permanente to discover what actually happened to patient care if we changed prescription drug coverage for a sizable population of our senior members in one large community. We changed our prescription drug benefits for 160,000 seniors, and then we tracked the impact of that benefit change on the senior patients affected.[70]

I want to be very clear about this entire process. We didn't change the prescription drug benefits to set up the research study. We changed benefits to keep total rates lower for that particular population of seniors. We moved from a full benefit prescription drug package to a $1,000 prescription drug benefit cap to reduce premiums charged to those seniors. The benefit cap saved premium dollars. But once a senior had used $1,000 worth of drugs, the drug benefit ended and those seniors had to pay for any additional drugs on their own. Since we were making that change and since we had a lot of good information about both the prior drug use of those seniors and about the way other members used their full-benefits packages, we decided to do a study to see exactly what impacts on people's health status and overall health care expenses that particular change in drug benefits might have. Keep in mind that the drug benefit cap was the only change. Everything else stayed exactly the same. The patients were in our care system seeing our doctors and going to our hospitals. The actual drug formulary was exactly the same. The only change was the new drug benefit cap. It was an almost perfect single variable study.

What did we learn? We learned not to use that approach. We learned that 18 percent of seniors who went over their $1,000 drug benefit started skipping doses of blood pressure medicine. Most of the people who stopped using the drugs were chronic care patients. That makes sense because chronic care patients use a lot of drugs.

Within twelve months, we saw a 9 percent increase in emergency room visits for those patients. We also saw a 13 percent increase in the hospital admission rate, and we actually saw a 22 percent increase in the mortality rate. Changing and reducing the drug coverage for seniors with chronic conditions increased other expenses for those seniors significantly within twelve months. More seniors were hospitalized, and more died. We don't know what the impact would have been in twenty-four months and thirty-six months, because we got rid of that benefit package. We do know, however, that the trend lines toward higher hospital use were pretty clear, so we expect that the negative hospital use consequences would have been worse in future years.

We stopped that coverage and we do not offer it anymore. Our researchers published the study in the *New England Journal of Medicine* on June 1, 2006.[71]

You can see other studies done by other organizations that show similar results.[72] It makes perfect sense. Deductibles are used exactly because they are intended to reduce the amount of care that people are willing to use. People who have to pay for prescriptions with their own out-of-pocket cash are less likely to fill them. The impact on higher-income people is tiny, but the impact on lower-income people is significant. A working single mother with a low income and three kids is not likely to follow the needed asthma protocols for her child with asthma if the office visits cost $100, the pulmonary function tests cost $80, and a couple of inhalers cost $200.

That can be a lot of money for someone who is paying rent, making a car payment, buying food, and buying clothes for a family.

Cost Sharing That Works

Some early studies of medical savings account products showed very little change in prescription refills for the people who voluntarily chose those products. That made perfect sense. When the products were entirely voluntary and offered to well-paid people who could estimate relatively well in advance what their out-of-pocket care costs would probably be, then the fact that well-paid people decided to use their tax-advantaged dollars to continue to refill their needed prescriptions shouldn't surprise anyone. The real test of the impact of these kinds of programs on people's care decisions is when the high-deductible products are not optional, but mandatory, and when low-income people with no money to save find themselves facing that same high-deductible benefit set.

That isn't to say that cost sharing, done well, is not a good idea. It can be a very good idea. Putting cost sharing in place for truly optional care decisions makes a lot of sense.

Having people pay more for brand-name drugs than for generic drugs makes a lot of sense.

Having percentage coinsurance plans that require the patients to pay 10 percent of a hospital stay for each day the patient spends in the hospital makes people aware of relative hospital costs. Also, that approach encourages patients to want to go home in five days rather than stay six or seven days. Hospital cost sharing can make a lot of sense, unless the income levels of the patient are really low.

But deliberately having people with significant chronic care needs financially incented not to buy needed medication makes less sense.

And people with lowest incomes are most likely to be adversely affected by extensive cost sharing. It's well documented that they skip care because they can't afford it.[73]

Equity issues aside, the real point to consider is that we can't succeed in bringing down the overall costs of care unless we deal more effectively with our chronic care patients—and our ability to deal more effectively with that 10 percent of our patient population who uses 70 percent of our costs is potentially impaired if the costs of preventive treatment keep them from participating in the preventive care patterns we need.

Congress definitely needs to resolve the issue of how to encourage—not discourage—use of appropriate prescriptions by chronic care patients when it next looks at the whole topic of consumer-directed care. The government now somewhat arbitrarily limits allowable up-front benefits for federally qualified medical savings accounts. As currently designed, those plans directly discourage sensible and needed care plans for our chronically ill patients. Those accounts should be set up to help us deal more effectively with chronic care treatment needs, not create barriers to those needs.

Solving the Chronic Disease Problem Doesn't Require Magic

The point of this chapter is that there are basic, productive, and systematic things we can do to reduce costs and improve care for the people with chronic disease who run up most of our health care costs.

Solving the cost problem for the top five chronic conditions doesn't require magic or a spectacular new program. It requires basic, consistent application of well-known facts of medical science and health care delivery. It requires consistent follow-up. It requires constant and systematic performance tracking to see which caregivers are delivering appropriate care and which patients are receiving appropriate care. It takes a system to get a systematic result.

If we stay focused and if we stay in constant problem-solving mode, we can get that job done—and everyone will benefit.

But we need a market environment that encourages and rewards best practices and that discourages and underfunds less-than-adequate practices in order for our care environment to function at optimal levels.

A number of recent developments have created an environmental change that could help put that new market in place. What are those changes?

Read on.

5

Eight Developments That Finally Make Health Care Reform Possible

Major health care reform is achievable right now in this country to a degree that literally was not possible until now.

Why do I say that? Because there are eight recent developments in American health care that have combined to give us, for the first time ever, a very real opportunity to systematically improve both care delivery and reduce the costs of care on a large scale in a relatively short time frame. I have touched on several of these issues in the prior chapters already. But I think we need to look at them as a package of events, opportunities, and issues that, taken together, give us a chance to make a real difference in American health care.

Those eight developments are creating what might be a "perfect storm" in favor of health care reform.

Without those specific developments, care delivery improvement and real market reform would be extremely difficult, if not impossible. With them, if we do the right things in the most effective ways, health care reform can actually happen. Soon.

So what are the magical eight recent developments that make health care reform much more possible right now?

1. Common Provider Number

The first key new health care reform ingredient is the common provider number. All health care providers in America will soon have, by law, a single identification number that clearly identifies each individual provider for all payers and for all care. That new single ID requirement is a huge step forward for health care data use.

The national single provider code requirement is a recent development, created by an extension of the Health Insurance Portability and Accountability Act of 1996 (HIPAA). This particular HIPAA provision requires use of the common provider number by May of 2007.[1]

The common provider number is an extremely important new tool. It changes access to care data in a critically important way. Until now, it has been functionally impossible to track individual provider performance using available electronic databases about care. The only electronic databases that exist have been created and held by the various payers of claims—the health plans, insurers, third party administrators, and public program payment shops. Each of these private and public payers has used its own unique, proprietary provider coding system, so there has been no way to link data from the various payers' claims payment databases in ways that could create either overall provider accountability or performance measurement. A single provider could and did have multiple identification codes, each code limited to a single payer's database, so the various payer databases could not be coordinated or aggregated in any effective way.

Tracking how well a given provider did in taking care of a chronic disease like asthma was made extremely difficult, if not impossible, by the fact that no two existing electronic records of his or her care could be linked together.

If we really believe that data is the essential first step for any continuous improvement process or model, then the importance of having a single, unique longitudinal numerical code for each provider becomes glaringly obvious. Health care reform becomes possible when we have real performance data about care.

2. Computerized Databases

The second major development that makes systematic health care reform finally possible is the emergence of computerized databases for all payers. Until very recently, a minority of health care claims were submitted electronically from care providers to insurers, health plans, and government payers. The resultant nonelectronic data flows were inconsistent and undependable in ways that significantly undermined the potential effectiveness of the final data sets for use in tracking health care delivery.

Today, with HIPAA regulations making the electronic data flow from providers to payers a standardized, more efficient, confidentially protected process, the databases for the payers are pretty much all electronic. The new HIPAA and industry standards for electronic data transmission also are set up to create a more uniform data flow.[2] As a result, the old, relatively inaccurate, and inefficient paper claim is being replaced very rapidly by far more accurate electronic claims submissions.

To make the process even more useful, the time frames between actual care delivery for a given patient and the electronic filing of a claim about that patient's incident of care have recently shrunk precipitously, to the point where the new electronic database for payers now has increasing value as a relatively current care management and provider support tool, as well as a history-based performance tracking tool.

3. Electronic Claims Data Portability

The value of that claims payment–based electronic data reporting tool is being further enhanced by the new willingness of the health care payer industry to commit as an entire industry to both data portability and data interoperability. The industry set itself a major new and almost revolutionary goal in 2006 to achieve a functional ability on the part of all insurers and payers to electronically move data between payers in ways that closely resemble comparable data flows in the banking industry. That ability is being piloted even as you are reading this book. So a significant supply of health care data is now becoming electronic, timely, standardized, and portable.

That is a data bonanza for health care. We are going from all data being held exclusively in separate paper medical records—inert and inaccessible—or in a myriad of fragmented electronic claims payment files with different data standards and unusable provider ID codes—to a new world of interchangeable electronic data and consistent, national provider ID codes. From a data perspective, that is revolutionary. It's a huge change.

There are, as I noted earlier, two major potential users for that new data. That new data flow can create longitudinal databases for each individual patient in the form of a personal health record, and it can also create communitywide databases that can be used to track patterns of care and caregiver performance.

Pulling electronic claims payment data out of paper-based insurance company files and making it available for measurable process improvement is a huge step forward for health care reform. We are at the first stages of that process, but I expect it to unfold very quickly once the database is available.

Again, the very best, most complete, and most useful database about patient care is the electronic medical record. The number of providers putting those complete automated medical record systems in place is growing rapidly. But many smaller provider sites are still several years away from having those full electronic medical record systems operational. In the meantime, however, as I described in earlier chapters, a lot of heavy lifting on health care accountability and reform can be done using the new electronic database created by the claims payment process and facilitated by HIPAA, the single provider ID number, and the new industry accords on data portability.

4. Governmental Transparency About Payment Data

A fourth major new element that enables and encourages reform is the unprecedented recent willingness of the government to create much greater levels of transparency about provider performance data using information from the current Medicare and Medicaid databases. The government has historically been both relatively secretive and extremely selective in its use of that data. The current administration is calling for a broad and sweeping transparency—a new level of data sharing from the government that could quickly prime the pump for important comparisons of provider performance.

In an executive order of August 22, 2006, the White House stated the following:

> It is the purpose of this order to ensure that health care programs administered or sponsored by the Federal Government promote quality and efficient delivery of health care through the use of health information technology, transparency regarding health care quality and price, and better incentives for program beneficiaries, enrollees, and providers. It is the further purpose of this order to make relevant information available to these beneficiaries, enrollees, and providers in a readily useable manner and in collaboration with similar initiatives in the private sector and non-Federal public sector.[3]

That is another revolutionary development. Medicare is the largest single purchaser of care in America.[4] To make that massive Medicare database about provider performance transparent is a huge step toward real market reform. That work isn't done yet, but it is now underway, and the enlightened intentions of the senior policymakers are pretty clear.

5. Universal Awareness of the Quality Issues

The fifth major development that is making health care reform possible now is the emergence, finally, of a widespread awareness across policymakers, politicians, buyers, care providers, and patients that our current health care infrastructure is badly flawed, perversely incented, inadequately coordinated, incredibly inconsistent, strategically unfocused, and too often dangerously dysfunctional. The powerful and persuasive Institute of Medicine studies combined with John Wennberg's work at Dartmouth and Beth McGlynn's work at RAND have shown beyond any doubt that our health care delivery infrastructure nonsystem leaves a lot to be desired.[5]

Until recently, quite a few health care policymakers wanted to restructure health care to get back to some level of entirely mythical "good old days"—the days when Marcus Welby–like physicians knew everything about care and made great, science-based decisions for each patient with no interference from any outside influences like health plans, government regulations, or scientific, performance-tracking databases.

Now, everyone knows that the world of unstructured care has given us a real quality chasm to cross—and a lot of people are ready for someone to design and build a bridge across that chasm. People are ready for some level of reform.

As I noted in the last chapter, a number of recent reformers have believed and hoped that if patients had to pay part of the bill then somehow—with no actual performance data of any kind—those patients would be able to make important decisions about caregivers in ways that would reward the best caregivers and introduce real market forces to health care. That theory is turning out to have some shortcomings. Deductibles obviously do not magically create data. Even when financially incented, uninformed consumers have a hard time making truly informed choices. That's the bad news.

There is also some very good news associated with that particular high-deductible benefit design experiment. One unintended positive consequence of testing those high-deductible plans was that people who wanted to make informed choices became very aware that they had no real information to use in making those choices.[6] People have begun to appreciate how little data patients have to make important care decisions.

People who know health care well now understand that those good old Marcus Welby days were an illusion and that the health care nonsystem we have today is too data-free, too often uncoordinated, too often outdated, usually badly structured, and even dangerous for far too many patients. The needs of the quality agenda for American health care are becoming very clear. Simply asking patients to make more choices won't create a marketplace based on best medical science. Buyers, patients, policymakers, and even care providers are all beginning to understand those realities.

The public trust has also been shaken by incidents like the Vioxx recall in 2004[7] and by a series of visible care direction missteps—like discovering that hormone replacement therapies for women did more harm than good[8] or that autologous bone marrow transplants for women with breast cancer made the death process more painful for the patients and added no length to those women's lives.[9]

So we have reached a point where large numbers of people are ready to look at change because there is a growing belief that the current pathway is both unaffordable and too often dysfunctional, or even unsafe.

Timing is everything. People are losing faith in the old quality agenda for care right at the point when a new agenda is possible.

6. Buyers Are Ready for a Change

In that vein, the sixth major factor that will accelerate the agenda for change is that the primary buyers of health care—the employers and government bodies who already purchase large quantities of health care—are now very ready for a change. It's hard to find a happy buyer. Companies look at how much their employees' and retirees' health care actually costs and they compare those costs to their competitors in other countries. For cars made in the United States, health care costs not only exceed the cost of steel—health care costs just for the retirees from American auto companies now exceed the cost of steel in each car. In 2005, GM spent $5.3 billion on health care; $4 billion covered retirees and their families.[10] Annual steel costs are about $3 billion.[11] The price tag of every GM car built in the United States includes $1,525 just for the health care of 1.1 million employees, retirees, and their families. Contrast this to the portion of a Toyota sticker price that accounts for health care: $97 for every vehicle built in Japan and $400 to $425 for each vehicle produced by Toyota in the United States.[12]

Buyers are ready for new answers. So are the government agencies that pay for government employees, as well as the government agencies that provide increasingly expensive health care to public program beneficiaries. This is actually a major sea change for the marketplace. It is needed.

Many employers over the past five to ten years have insisted that stricter versions of available cost containment approaches should not be applied to their employees—and many employers relatively recently refused to allow their health plans or benefit administrators to restrict access to certain providers and rejected proposals to channel patients to a select group of proven, cost-effective caregivers. Those particular buyer constraints are fast fading away, and buyers are now cutting benefits and imposing coverage eligibility restrictions. Many are now considering using more tightly managed care networks to significantly reduce costs. On a more drastic level, many buyers are now canceling or freezing health care coverage for their retirees and, sadly, large numbers of smaller employers are even dropping employee coverage all together. Less than half of all firms with fewer than ten workers now offer health benefits, compared to more than 90 percent of firms with fifty or more employees.[13]

It's a time of change for many buyers. Buyers are ready for new answers—answers that work. That readiness makes change possible. Markets and industries do not change when customers aren't ready to change. In this case, the buyers are now ready for change a bit before the vendors have figured out how to change. Reform will be possible when that happens. Vendors will, I expect, rise to the occasion. That's how markets work.

7. Internet Functionality Used for Care

The seventh major factor that is currently strongly enabling an environment of change in health care is the Internet. The Internet has already had a huge impact on other areas of the economy. Purchasing, banking, investing, and education are all areas where the Internet has made massive inroads into how we do business.

Health care is poised to follow. Health and medical web sites receive the highest number of visits from search engines.[14] As an evolving health care economy learns to use the Internet more effectively, we will soon see more doctor-patient e-connections. E-scheduling, e-visits, e-follow-ups and reports, and e-reminders about needed care all are rolling out now in various places.

The future scope and volume of e-visits and e-connections will, I believe, exceed almost everyone's expectations. Patients will have various kinds of innovative and easy-to-use testing equipment in their homes and will be making e-connections with their caregivers in multiple ways. The current explorations into supporting some levels of in-home care will, I believe, explode over the next several years as the population ages and the availability of some levels of face-to-face or institutional care become problematic.

That's a longer-term view. The short-term view involves a lot of Internet use fairly quickly.

The new market model for health care will rely heavily on the Internet, as patients both choose real live caregivers based on e-data and then get quick and convenient electronic advice about their care from e-consultants. The very best versions of the new market model will rely on the Internet to get information to patients and to caregivers and to facilitate patient choices relative to caregivers, care strategies, care plans, and actual care. Only the computer can facilitate those levels of choices in any workable way. A paper-based, data-rich health care marketplace would be logistically crippled. Paper can't do the job. We need the web to reform care.

Also, when all patients have electronic personal health records (PHRs) available on the Internet from their payers—and when the PHRs have each patient's diagnosis, tests, prescriptions, and lists of each and every care procedure performed for each patient by each caregiver—patients will be able to plug that electronic PHR information into e-consults, getting virtual second opinions from medical experts in the computerized care business who will be obsessively up-to-date on the best available care options for each diagnosis.

The Internet will make medical science more current. Individual doctors in individual practices may currently have a hard time keeping up with each new scientific development in their specialty, but the new companies and care providers who will sell their services on the Internet to provide e-consults will consider keeping up with current science a key value they sell to patients. It will transform care when people with asthma bring e-consult printouts to their real-life, in-the-flesh caregivers to ask why a particular drug is or is not being used for their care.

The e-consults will say, "You have asthma. You have been in the emergency room three times this year. There are three good drugs that might be used at this point. Here's a list of these drugs and their normal retail prices. You seem to be using the most expensive of those three drugs now. You could save $120 a month by switching to the least expensive drug. Here's the most recent comparative test data about the relative effectiveness of each of those drugs. Do you have any questions?"

Some very bad medical service is now provided over the web. Current health care web sites may be credible or may be charlatans. My sense is that an industry of credible sites will emerge as an option for many patients.

Even the credible independent e-consultant firms that will be on the web probably would run into real local license problems if they actually tried to practice free-standing Internet medicine. However, those businesses would probably have relatively easy sailing if they simply shared care protocols, pointed out where current treatment for a given patient differed from those protocols, and then suggested that the patient discuss care options directly with her primary caregiver. Since most primary caregivers will be handling e-inquiries from their own patients over the next several years, the medical issue question-and-answer process for some patients might be entirely electronic, from the patient to the e-consultant through to the live local physicians and then back to the patients.

That level of very direct e-dialogue with patients has the potential to significantly impact the delivery of care. It definitely has the potential to significantly shorten the seventeen-year time frame that the IOM noted is often the length of time before a new best care approach is uniformly used by all physicians.[15]

The Internet by itself will help educate people about their medical conditions and their care. The Internet combined with personal health records, virtual consults, and extensive comparative performance data about various caregivers will probably revolutionize some aspects of care.

Couple that functionality with e-visits, e-dialogue, and direct patient e-connectivity with his chosen caregiver or care-teams, and it's easy to see how health care reform could—and will—be significantly e-impacted.

The best care systems will offer e-connectivity to their patients in ways not even dreamed of today. E-visits will be an expectation, a basic level of patient-provider interaction that will allow for whole new levels of care convenience and care growth. Health care will be an e-industry relatively soon.

8. Lawmakers Are Ready for Reform

The final new development that will allow real health care reform to happen is the fact that lawmakers in a great many states have also hit the tipping point on the need for real care reform.

State legislative budgets are being destroyed by the increasing costs of care. Emergency rooms are closing, and inner-city hospitals are imperiled. The number of uninsured Americans continues to grow, and the number of underinsured Americans may be growing even faster as high-deductible health plans increase in number.[16] Too many of the purely uninsured people do not vote, so it's far too easy for elected officials not to hear their voices.

Underinsured Americans—people who are insured but face out-of-pocket costs that are high relative to their incomes[17]—can, however, create a major new political backlash because the underinsured tend to be fully employed people,[18] who are more likely to vote.[19] Underinsured people vote and they are getting angry. When enough are angry, they will be heard.

So state after state is now aiming at some kind of health care reform, usually targeted at the twin goals of increasing the number of insured people while cutting costs (see Exhibit 5.1).

So far, there has been a major shortage of proposals that can meet both those goals of increasing the number of insured while cutting costs, but the momentum across the country to pass legislation of some kind shouldn't be underestimated. Leaders in legislatures and governors' mansions are ready to act, as are labor unions and major employers—once a solid course of action becomes clear.

So buyers are ready, labor unions are ready, consumers are ready, politicians are ready, academics are ready, and even some caregivers

Exhibit 5.1. State Health Insurance and Universal Coverage Initiatives.

Universal Health Care. At least twenty states have introduced related legislation: California, Colorado, Connecticut, Florida, Hawaii, Kansas, Illinois, Maine, Maryland, Massachusetts, Minnesota, Missouri, New Hampshire, New York, Ohio, Oklahoma, Pennsylvania, Rhode Island, Vermont, and Wisconsin.

The following are examples of legislation relating to universal health care:

Maine	Dirigo Health Reform Act: coverage for every citizen by 2009
Illinois	All Kids Health Insurance Program: all children under the age of eighteen can access coverage if not covered by family policies or state-sponsored programs
Massachusetts	Chapter 58 of the Acts of 2006: every person in the Commonwealth will have health care access by 2009
Vermont	Health Care Affordability Act: creates Catamount Health to provide affordable, comprehensive coverage for residents

Mandated Employer Health Insurance Coverage. At least fourteen states have introduced related legislation: Kansas, Kentucky, Massachusetts, Michigan, Minnesota, New Jersey, New York, Ohio, Oregon, Pennsylvania, Rhode Island, Tennessee, Washington, West Virginia.

One state has enacted legislation requiring employers to provide health insurance coverage:

Massachusetts	Creates a "fair share contribution" for employers that do not offer health insurance to their employees and imposes a "free rider surcharge" on employers who don't provide health insurance and whose employees use free care.

are ready. We now have the potential of a new electronic database that could serve as the foundation for systematically improving many areas of care. How do we get those eight developments to merge into a single agenda to reform care?

An Optimal Health Care Market

Let's revisit one more time what an optimal health care marketplace might look like. As business guru Stephen Covey says, "Begin with the end in mind."[20] What do we want to see in our care delivery system?

- *Consumers should have complete and easy electronic access to their own health information*. Patients should be able to find which medications they have been prescribed, which doctors they have seen recently, and which procedures they have had done over their lifetimes. It's amazing, but consumers don't have an easy way to access this information now.
- *Consumers should have complete and easy electronic access to the information they need to make informed decisions about their caregivers*. A patient needing knee surgery should have data available to figure out which surgeons are most likely to achieve a satisfactory result. A patient with asthma should know which teams of caregivers are most likely to manage the disease successfully and help the patient avoid the asthma attacks that undermine the patient's quality of life and sometimes threaten life itself.
- *Consumers should have complete and easy electronic access to the information they need to make informed decisions about their care*. A patient with heart disease should be able to find out what complications others have experienced from bypass surgery. Patients with asthma should know what drugs are available to best treat their particular triggers. Patients should have the opportunity to get consultations electronically about various approaches appropriate for their care.

Ideally, consumers should be empowered and educated, supported and encouraged in receiving best care and in making the lifestyle choices that support their own best possible personal health.

Care should be accessible and affordable, with patients having enough appropriate involvement in the cost of care to encourage wise choices by the patients and competitive prices by the caregivers.

Consumers should be able to have confidence that their own caregivers are current relative to medical science and best care and obsessively conscientious about the follow-up needed for their care.

It's not hard to figure out what the ideal health care marketplace might look like. The challenge is to actually make it happen. Someone needs to actually provide the data flow processes and communication infrastructures needed for patients to make those informed choices. The pieces can all be assembled from available components. The need is for a market model that will reward the vendors who can functionally make that infrastructure happen.

The next chapter deals with why market forces have not worked well in health care up to now. Chapter Seven then suggests a new market model that might work to actually meet our needs for a better system.

For now, the point I'd like to make is that the emergence of a single provider number, electronic personal health records, data portability, and a sense by key parties that change is really needed all work together to set up the best environment and opportunity we've ever had for real health care reform in America. We just need to be very clear on what that reform should be. And we should be clear that we need that reform now.

6

Making the Market Work for Health Care

One of the most common questions asked by both health care policymakers and health care purchasers is, "Why don't market forces have the same impact on health care that they have in just about every other area of our economy?" The follow-up question that is asked almost as often is, "Why does computerization reduce costs in other areas of the economy and not in health care?"

Those are both great questions. They both have very simple answers. The short answer to the first question is that market forces actually do have a very powerful impact every single day on health care structure, delivery, and performance in this country. We get exactly what we pay for and we get more of that than any health care economy in the world. We just pay too often for the wrong stuff. We need to set up carefully structured incentives that reward our care infrastructure in a useful and persuasive way for performing in a manner that will improve both care quality and care efficiency. This chapter will offer a few thoughts about how that might be done. Health care can be restructured using market incentives—we just need to use the right incentives and target them very well.

The second question is, "Why haven't computers cut costs in health care like they have in every other area of the economy?" That answer is also fairly simple and it is tied directly to the first answer. Computers haven't cut costs in health care because providers are not rewarded today for cutting costs. Cutting overall health care costs is not an overarching goal for fee-for-service caregivers, so obviously very few fee-for-service health care organizations or professionals are trying to figure out how to use computers to achieve that nonexistent goal. Follow the money trail. Using computers, for example, to cut the overall costs of heart care will only reduce total provider revenue for heart patients, with no increase in patient volume or caregiver profitability to make up for the revenue loss. We know from pilot studies that computer support tools can help lower the rate of heart attacks to a third below average.[1] But almost no one is rewarded for cutting those costs, so that's not how the vast majority of caregiver computers are used. Computers will be used very well in a great many ways to cut health care costs as soon as the health care market model actually directly rewards providers for cutting those costs.

An Ideal Health Care Marketplace

If we want a new value-based, appropriately incented health care marketplace to exist, someone has to make it happen. Before we can set up a market model with incentives to produce the care product we want, we need to spend a little time defining what that new health care product might be. Let me offer a couple of thoughts in that regard: in an ideal health care marketplace, the best caregivers would be recognized for their skill and achievements and be rewarded both financially and professionally for their accomplishments. In an ideal health care world, patients could make fully informed choices about their caregivers and their care—and individual consumers and patients who act in responsible ways to improve and maintain their own health should and would benefit from those efforts.

An ideal health care world would be based on the best available science, the best array of informed choices, and it should be affordable to all participants. The ideal health care world would cover everyone, with no one left uninsured or without needed care. In an ideal health care world, market forces would be fully engaged, with those market forces aimed strategically at achieving a health care marketplace of excellence, efficiency, and informed choice.

That can, I believe, all be done—but only if we carefully design the desired health care marketplace and only if key buyers then decide to use that new marketplace to purchase their care.

The Buyer's Role Is Critical

The role of buyers is critical. Each and every area of the economy responds directly to the incentives and opportunities presented by its buyers. Think about how the market actually works for other industries. Retail sales, for example, are heavily market-based. Buyers in the retail world reward products that meet their needs by actually buying those products. Buying is the key step. Manufacturers design and produce the products that are actually purchased. Buyers purchase cell phones with certain features, so those cell phones are manufactured. Buyers buy television sets with certain features, so those TVs are made. Made and sold. Televisions that aren't purchased are no longer manufactured. To an extreme degree. It's pretty hard to find a black-and-white television these days. No one buys them, so no one makes them.

Health care is no exception. We reward imaging services, so America is second only to Japan in the number of MRI machines per citizen.[2] The percentage of health care spending that goes to diagnostic imaging is growing at a pace that exceeds almost anything else in health care.[3] An MRI is purely a cost center in Canada, an expense paid for painfully out of taxpayers' dollars in the context of a tightly controlled provincial budget. So the number of MRI machines in Canada is limited and scans are done less often.[4]

In the United States, MRIs are paid for on a per-use basis—not through a fixed and limited budget—and the use fee in the United States is generally quite profitable for whoever owns the machine. So the total cost and use of imaging in the United States is a multiple of the cost in Canada—U.S. $100 billion for imaging costs in the United States versus U.S. $2 billion in Canada[5]—and those costs are still growing in this country at a pace that exceeds almost anything else in health care. Only Japan has more MRI machines than we do and, as any good economist might have guessed, the owners of those Japanese machines are also paid on a fee-for-service basis. Figure 6.1 depicts these relationships.

Market forces are clearly at work. The market in this country directly rewards imaging, so we get a lot of images. The good news is that the new imaging technology really does provide doctors

Figure 6.1. Diagnostic Imaging Units per Million Population.

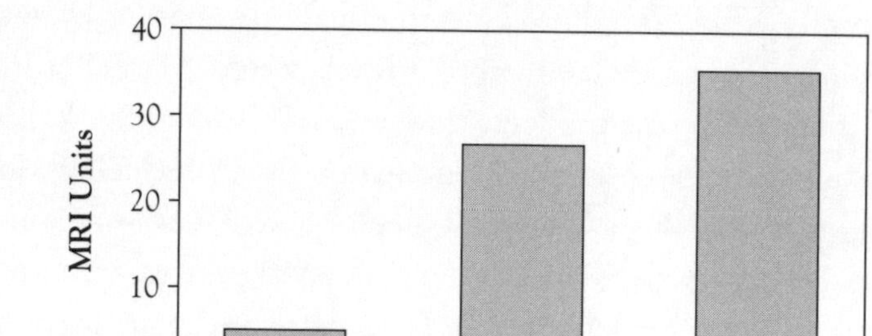

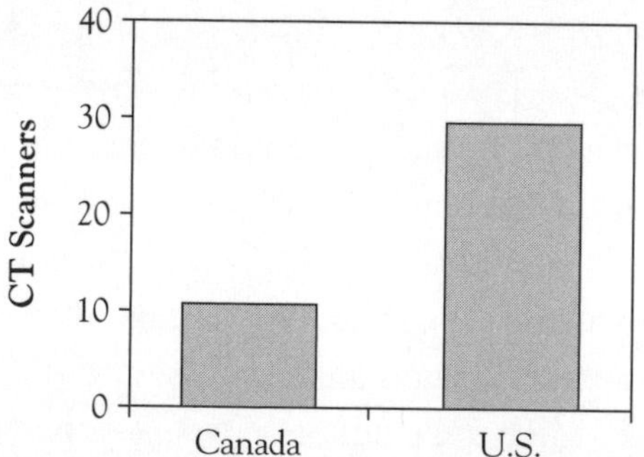

Source: Organisation for Economic Co-operation and Development. "OECD Health Data 2006: Frequently Requested Data." Oct. 10, 2006. http://www.oecd.org/document/16/0,2340en_2825_495642_2085200_1_1_1_1,00.html.

with a wonderful diagnostic tool. Imaging is a growing science and it truly is a great tool for improving the quality of care. Some of the diagnoses made by imaging equipment could not be made in any other way. Also, we always need to keep in mind that the only alternative to some specific imaging techniques is exploratory surgery.

Speaking directly from a patient quality-of-life perspective, getting scanned is almost always a lot better than getting cut. It's particularly good when the cut would otherwise need to be made deep in an organ—or worse yet, inside the brain. So scans can be very good. The bad news is that quite a few diagnoses that use expensive imaging equipment could have been made equally well with a lot less expense, using expertise and other less costly tests. The profitability of imaging in this country definitely impacts its use levels.

Likewise, specialists get paid a lot of money, so we have more specialists in America than anywhere else in the world by a significant margin. Primary care providers in America tend to be less well paid, so we are on the verge of a shortage of primary care physicians. Many internal medicine teaching residencies are currently in danger of being underenrolled. Family practice residencies in the United States are currently filled by just 41 percent of students educated in U.S. medical schools.[6] American medical students just are not interested in becoming family practitioners. By contrast, specialist residencies like dermatology and plastic surgery are 80 percent filled with students educated in U.S. medical schools.[7]

Again, market forces are at work. Buyers now reward specialty and subspecialty services with high fees and no substantive questions about outcomes, so expensive specialty care is exactly what we get. See Figure 6.2 to understand why American medical students are motivated to become specialists.

So financial incentives do significantly influence American health care today. Health care is sculpted by those incentives. Incentives work. We just need to do a better job of figuring out what to incent. The relevant economic theory is pretty simple.

Figure 6.2. Annual Compensation of Physicians in Selected Primary Care and Specialty Practices.

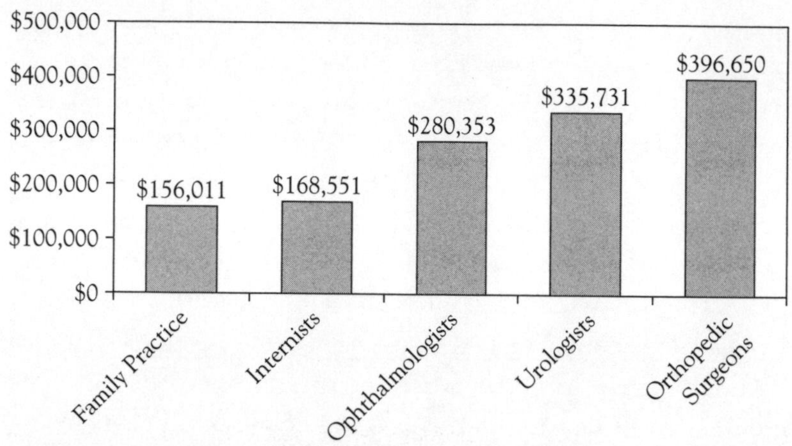

Source: Medical Group Management Association. "Specialty Group Practice Physicians' Compensation Stagnates," news release, Aug. 31, 2005; C. Pope, "Orthopedic Surgeon's Compensation Slips a Bit." MGMA *e-Connexion*, Nov. 2005, vol. 88.

To create a health care delivery system in this country designed for optimal efficiency, optimal quality, and optimal accessibility, we basically need to (1) set up an economic model that rewards each of those desired outcomes, and then (2) we need to use it. An economic system with no buyers dies a quick death. An economic system with a lot of buyers thrives.

Rhetoric will not make health care reform and a new market model happen. Wishful thinking will not make it happen. We need buyers to demand this kind of reform and then buy it. The new economic model for health care has to be used and purchased in volume, or it will never become a reality. Market forces need to be used with cash attached in order to have any real-world impact on the actual delivery of care.

That is elementary economics, but it's a point of fact that has been pretty much ignored in the health care policy debate up to this point. A few innovative thinkers, like professor Alain Enthoven from Stanford,[8] the architect of the managed competition model of health care reform, have proposed very workable market models to improve both the efficiency and quality of care, but these models have not been refined and, sadly, they have been only sporadically used. When used, they worked.

The Government Would Have Trouble Setting Up the Market

The U.S. government is one of the major purchasers of health care: over 40 percent of health care costs are paid by government agencies. (See Chapter Ten for a full explanation of the government's role as a purchaser of health care.) There are certainly defined roles for government in the market reform proposal outlined in this book, both for creating an enabling legal context for some aspects of the new market and then for purchasing care and mandating transparency about that care. I do not believe, however, that the government can or should be the main instrument of initial market reform if what we want is a viable, flexible, innovating marketplace of competing providers of care.

If the government tries to set up all of the specifics and operational details of a new provider competition marketplace, the results are likely to be a bit more rigid than we need. In a worst-case situation, if we used the government to set up the new, interprovider market infrastructure, we could end with a messy, ineffective, and potentially crippling mixture of partisan politics, economic special-interest lobbying, and the normal operational and logistical constraints of traditional bureaucracy. We would need a consensus model if the government is at its core.

Building consensus in a governmental setting is not easy. Bringing together a wide range of interests is a solid process that definitely has its place in the context of governing a democratic country, but it is not quick or easy to do.

If the developmental process for governmental policy in a democracy is done well, it will be inherently political. We are truly blessed by living in a democratic form of government, where all voices can be heard—some better than others. In an optimal and equitable political model, all interested parties would be heard and the ultimate result of the decision-making process would tend to be the product of a melded consensus. That consensus-based decision-making approach can be wonderful, and it can also have some shortcomings. When we try to be creative by consensus, decisions on key issues too often default to a complex meld of various public interests and special interests all influencing the process through various lobbying efforts and through targeted campaigns of direct public and policymaker persuasion. Everyone in that kind of process is generally given a chance to provide input—usually multiple times in multiple settings—but the people who are heard the most may have interests not optimally aligned with the cause of true reform.

Our complex, multilayered, time-consuming American democratic process has the wonderful usual and customary consequence of almost always keeping short-sighted and dictatorial governmental whims of the moment from becoming American public policy. Leaders don't typically create major programs in America or take us in truly new directions by sheer use of power. It's hard to stampede American lawmaking in any given direction. That's generally a very good thing—but, to repeat myself just a bit, it also makes crisp and immediate reform in any area highly unlikely. If we truly want crisp and quick reform, we need to engage the private marketplace, not the regulatory infrastructure.

We actually very much need the government to do some heavy lifting to help move the reform process along. But my point is we probably do not want the government, with all its layers and complexities, to be the key central agent of change. We need buyers—expert and highly motivated buyers—to be the key agents for initial change.

Consumers as Buyers

As I noted earlier, payers have been experimenting with some market model changes by modifying insurance benefit packages in ways that place a heavier up-front financial burden on individual insured persons for the costs of their initial care. The theory and hope was that the new benefit packages would cause individual buyers—consumers—to make better decisions about their care.

That line of thought is a small but encouraging step in a generically good direction. The good direction is that a number of people are obviously ready to develop a strategy of some kind to selectively use market forces in health care. But, as discussed earlier in this book, the actual financial incentives used to influence patient behavior with that specific initial theoretical benefit design were a little crude, a bit blunt, and, in the real world, too often more than a little counterproductive—particularly relative to the care needs of the chronic care patients who create our major cost burden.

So the good news is that there is an increasing tendency and willingness on the part of payers to use market forces to help reform care. The bad news is that the specific economic tools that have been proposed up to this point are clearly inadequate for the full scope of the economic heavy lifting that needs to be done. The best elements of these ideas need to be incorporated into a more comprehensively designed approach that actually could improve care quality, care efficiency, health care choices, and access to care.

Major Buyers Need to Take the Lead

The private sector—represented most effectively by the major employers who already purchase health coverage for the majority of our citizens and whose direct health coverage contributions now total roughly 26 percent of the total health care dollars spent in America[9]—are the folks most likely to achieve, refine, and deploy a successful new market model for the country. The government, as a buyer, should be a fast follower, once a new market model is shown to work. Once it is proven to work, the government could use the new model to provide coverage and care first to government employees, and then to the people covered by our various entitlement programs. Medicare and Medicaid should be part of the overall reform agenda as soon as that new marketplace takes root.

Large private employers are the best choice for implementing the new market model for a couple of reasons. One is that many large employers are already highly skilled purchasers for everything else they purchase. So becoming highly skilled purchasers for health care is a logical extension of their current skill set. A second reason for believing the major employers should drive this agenda is that major employers already have a lot at stake relative to health care costs.[10] We looked at some of those numbers earlier. The costs for American employers of buying care already far exceed the health care costs borne by their competitors from other countries. U.S. employers pay an average of $6,600 per year per employee; their Canadian counterparts, for instance, pay only about $600 a year.[11] Our employers have significant economic skin in the game now, so to speak, and are—as they say in real estate circles—already highly motivated buyers.

The third reason is flexibility. The government inherently has a hard time being either flexible or creative. As noted above, that isn't a bad thing, because we don't want a government for this country that zigs and zags from policy point to policy point on an irregular basis. Generic governmental policy inflexibility is the price we Americans pay for stability. It's usually a fair price to pay. Stability can be a good thing. After you've seen a few other countries firsthand where the government can more easily zig and zag based on the ideology of the moment and the dictatorship of the current majority, it's easier to more fully appreciate the value of our American governmental stability. But that stability means that we need to use another leverage factor to achieve initial health care reform—using market forces as a critical component. The very best market forces, as I noted, can and will come from highly motivated private buyers. So how can that be done?

Let's take a deeper look at how market forces affect other aspects of our economy. It's a useful exercise in what market forces can and cannot do.

We Need Both Retail and Wholesale Market Forces

In most other areas of the economy, market forces have an obvious and powerful impact on the costs of goods produced and sold. My experience is that computers, telephones, bedspreads, casual clothes, and even laundry detergent all cost less in 2006 than they did in 1996, and even with those lower prices the higher-tech products also are far better and more functional than the versions we had available a decade ago.

What has caused those other industries to continuously increase efficiency and reduce price, and what learnings can we bring from that success to health care?

For most of the items we buy, the market works at two levels: the wholesale level and the retail level. The two-level marketplace is an extremely important concept to understand. Wholesale buyers at Target, Wal-Mart, JCPenney, Sears, and other major retailers function as level one—the volume purchasers. The big volume purchasers have a lot of leverage. They insist on vendors continuously improving both their products and their prices. I've heard personally from the CEOs of several major product vendors for the big retailers how much pressure they feel and, in some cases, how much the vendors dislike the major wholesale buyers' constant pressures for both quality and lower price.

Wal-Mart may not be loved by all of its vendors, but it is loved by the Wal-Mart shoppers who pay less for a DVD player or a pair of Levi's in 2006 than they paid in 1996.[12] Why do they pay less? Only because the wholesale buyers at Wal-Mart use their leverage and expertise to keep that constant pressure on their vendors.[13] In a world of escalating expenses, Wal-Mart prices (and prices at Target, JCPenney, Best Buy, Sears, and so on) make the "good life" affordable for a lot of American consumers.

Vendors may not always like the pressure, but they benefit from those market forces as well if they can achieve the price and quality standards of the big buyers. The vendors who meet the cost and value standards of the major wholesale buyers benefit financially based on volume—they sell a lot of product because of their low prices. And their volume allows them to keep prices low. It's a cycle of consequences and rewards that works well for the consumer.

It's a mistake to underestimate the impact that those high-volume retailers have on the production of goods and products for consumer sales in America. If the major Wal-Mart and Target types of wholesale purchasers did not exist, the cost of pots, pans, bed linens, and color TVs would be a lot higher in this country. If we all bought our TVs solely from neighborhood stores that each sold very small numbers of TVs locally to a small set of customers, TVs would cost a lot more and they probably would do a lot less in terms of functionality. Maybe fewer TVs would be a good thing, depending on your personal perception of the community impact and the ethical and social value of ever-present television, but whatever your views it would be a lot more expensive to buy each TV unit if the economic pressure that we see today from the big wholesale purchasers did not exist.

That's the first major learning I believe health care economists need to look at—prices in other important and relevant markets are influenced downward by the role played by large, economically powerful, wholesale buyers who directly reward the specific vendors who achieve low costs. Those same wholesale buyers reject vendors with high costs. Health care right now does not have any entities functioning effectively as equivalent wholesale purchasers of entire health care products, so there is no current marketplace for complete health care products.

Health care needs organizations like Target, Best Buy, and Walmart—vendors who create a place where people buy and who insist that the direct suppliers who sell in those markets perform at acceptable levels and generate both quality products and good prices. Imagine a retail world without the big retailers. Then think about how much we need an equivalent market force in health care. I'll return to that point in a few pages.

Retail Sales Involve Individual Informed Choices

The second set of learnings for health care from the general marketplace is that retail sales made directly to consumers add another level of market forces that also work to improve product quality, value, and variety.

In most areas of the economy, consumers can make quite a few individual choices about the products they buy, choosing between brands and models based on individual consumer criteria. For large-ticket items like cars, appliances, and equipment, the individual consumer who makes a purchase often has quite a bit of objective performance and quality data and expert analysis easily available to help compare one product to another. Various car magazines, computer magazines, and web sites like *Consumer Reports* make comparative data on those products easily available to individual buyers. A person wanting to compare an Apple computer to a PC would be awash in various levels of comparative information about each product available to the interested consumer from their own home via the Internet. Product manufacturers in the retail marketplace are rewarded by customers making informed individual purchases. Products that appeal to a lot of individual purchasers win the sales war and therefore survive.

Market forces, in other words, shape participants through both the wholesale and retail marketplace. Wholesale and retail market forces combine to give us the marketplace we have for TV sets, gas dryers, winter coats, and jet skis. Health care, I believe, also needs to figure out how to use both wholesale and retail market models and functionality in order to simultaneously improve quality and reduce prices.

No Comparable Health Care Marketplace

Today there is no comparable health care marketplace. Individual consumers have little or no comparative data about product features, caregiver performance, or care. Major buyers simply do not function in health care like they do in purchasing computers at the wholesale level.

Right now, health care lacks both a set of wholesale buyers who can incent overall product costs and performance, and informed retail buyers who can make individual choices about health care vendors and services.

Remember, we've already shown pretty clearly that direct market forces are currently shaping the existing American health care infrastructure and marketplace. As noted in Chapter One, market forces actually are having a huge impact on care today. The market forces that exist in health care now are extremely powerful, but they are so badly structured that they lead to a marketplace that penalizes efficiency, encourages inconsistency, and has absolutely no demonstrable relationship between the price of any single health care product and its actual value. The market forces we have allowed to function in health care today have fed the growth of a massive health care cost structure, huge volumes of sometimes inappropriate and even dangerous services, and an extremely expensive array of unlinked, uncoordinated vendors selling individual, unconnected units of care, rather than selling actual care outcomes.

Think about it. You saw the numbers earlier. The current system has nine thousand billing codes for individual health care services, and not one single billing code for a cure. There is no payment for improved health. There's no financial reward for improved outcomes. There are instead massive payments—billions and billions of dollars paid—to more than a million caregivers for separate pieces of care.

So what do we get from that economic model? Cures at the most competitive price? Never. We get exactly what we pay for. The health care marketplace today does what every market does: it sells what people are buying and willing to pay for. We buy and pay for nine thousand services. So that's what we get.

We need market forces like the ones that can get us a better DVD player for less than half the prior cost and still generate a reasonable profit for the DVD manufacturer, not market forces that increase health care costs at double-digit levels every year while providing less than adequate care to half our population and leaving more than forty-five million Americans uninsured.

So how can more appropriate market forces be created in health care? It won't happen on its own. Nor is there a silver bullet solution.

We Need Infrastructure Vendors (IVs)

In order for market forces to reward desired provider performance, we need to identify first exactly what that desired performance is, and then we need to directly reward someone for achieving those results. That may seem pretty basic, but it's not the way some people have been thinking.

Market forces can, I believe, transform care, but not just any random, generic, or crude market forces. For market forces to directly transform care, we need to do more than put consumers at risk for the first dollar cost of care and then expect individual patients to somehow create rewards for the best providers. Even if one consumer or another somehow manages to make those kinds of caregiver selection decisions well, the informed choice leverage from one consumer is not likely to transform any single multimillion-dollar revenue provider of care into a more accountable vendor, much less create a whole marketplace full of accountable, efficient, low-cost vendors. Economic forces require scale and volume to have impact. Single consumer choices have no scale and therefore by themselves little impact.

So what can be done to apply market forces to improve the cost and quality of care? We need to hire a vendor to set up and administer those market forces. We need to deliberately use both wholesale purchasing leverage and retail purchasing leverage to make the care system more productive and individual providers more directly impacted by their performance and efficiency. We need to take the current, massive, unlinked, extremely expensive infrastructure of American health care and hire someone to change how that infrastructure performs.

We need infrastructure vendors—IVs for short—and we need those IVs to put in place the data gathering, tracking, and communication tools needed to reform health care delivery. The role of the IVs is an essential one. And only buyers can assign that needed role to the infrastructure reform vendors and then give them control over enough health care revenue flow to make reform real. That's the proposal outlined in the next chapter. It's a very different way of looking at how we Americans buy care—but it's the right way to buy care if what we want is efficient, accountable, high-quality, consumer-focused, continuously improving care.

So don't stop reading yet. More to come.

7

A New Idea: The Infrastructure Vendor

Given the critically important and highly influential role of the buyer, what exactly should major buyers do to change the way care is purchased and delivered in America?

At its core, this new market strategy calls for America's major buyers to purchase wisely. Purchasing wisely is not a new area of expertise for large companies. The truth is that every large company currently rates purchasing wisely as a major strategic agenda and as a core operational competency for its overall non–health care business.[1]

Car manufacturers purchase component parts for their cars all the time with a very high level of competency. The specifications for purchasing hubcaps extend to a thousandth, even millionths, of an inch, to the actual molecular composition of the hubcap material, and to error rates and delivery times for the hubcaps production process. Clothing manufacturers purchase buttons and thread using solid comparative and competitive market data, product testing, and highly detailed quality compliance standards.

Health care purchasing has not been held to similar standards. But when we have reached the point where the cost of health care at GM exceeds the cost of steel in a car and the cost of health care coverage at Starbucks exceeds the actual cost of coffee, then it's time for the major buyers to stop thinking of health care as a cost-plus, unengineered, externally shaped, seller-defined, completely unmanaged purchasing expense. It's time for buyers to subject health care to the same kind of detailed performance expectations or specifications as they use for their core business products, and to introduce a whole new level of expertise and leverage into the purchase of both health care coverage and health care delivery.

How can that most easily be done? The key to health care reform in America using a market model will be for the buyers to hire infrastructure vendors (IVs) to set up the needed marketplace. The new marketplace will not exist until someone is hired to make it happen, so we need vendors who can transform the infrastructure and performance of care in clearly defined ways. These IVs will function in part as the wholesalers that the health care marketplace currently lacks for certain levels of health care services—they will be the Best Buys, Targets, and Wal-Marts of health care. Health care providers will create the actual care delivery product. The IVs will be the wholesalers, setting up the megastore-equivalent environment that will be the context for individual consumers purchasing care and for care providers selling care. The IVs will also contract with health care providers for care and will help the providers create care packages for patients and employers that met the buyers' specifications. Employers will select the IVs that their employees will be able to use for their care delivery and care decisions and will create specifications for how the IVs will perform. Specifications are key. To make health care reform happen, major buyers will need to create an array of specifications for an integrated health care delivery, financing, and patient support infrastructure and then buy health care reform packages from skilled and well-run vendors who can satisfy those expectations.

What Should the New Marketplace Look Like?

Buyers need to clearly define what market enhancement services they want to buy. Buyers need to set up a proposal process and issue specifications and then hire vendors who can meet their specifications. Exactly what specifications should the buyers invoke and impose on their vendors to make that new marketplace appear and then perform?

Let me start by describing once again what an optimal market for health care would look like and do.

- An optimal health care marketplace would give consumers and patients informed choices about both caregivers and care. The IVs should create the needed data flow and process to make that happen.
- An optimal health care marketplace would use the techniques of systems thinking and process reengineering to continuously improve care outcomes and reduce the cost of care. The IVs should support the caregivers in making continuous process improvement a necessity and a reality and should present the results of those processes to the patients making choices about caregivers.
- An optimal health care marketplace would reward the best caregivers for being the best—and create a context, process, and set of incentives that would cause other caregivers to improve their performances as well. The IVs need to put that structure in place and demonstrate to the buyers that the process works.
- An optimal health care marketplace would provide access to needed care for all patients. The IVs can help achieve that goal (see Chapter Eleven for how).
- An optimal health care marketplace would be interconnected in multiple ways so that continuity of care would be a performance expectation easily met rather than the rare occurrence it now is, achieved with difficulty and created more often by lucky breaks rather than by systematic communication and well-engineered connectivity tool kits. The IVs should facilitate and operate electronic connectivity support tools for the patients and caregivers and should demonstrate their effectiveness to the buyers.
- An optimal health care marketplace would have incentives and supports built in for consumers to make wise choices about their

health care treatments and even wiser choices about their personal health status—with direct consumer accountability for their own personal health both encouraged and supported by the caregivers, the care system, the financial arrangements, the benefit designs, and the expectations of the overall care environment. The IVs should help with benefit designs that reinforce these goals and with extensive and systematic patient education and support tools to facilitate healthier behaviors.

In short, the optimal marketplace should be data-rich, strategically incented, ergonomically elegant, electronically interconnected, economically efficient, and set in a context of constant systems enhancement and process improvement. That's the environment the IVs should be hired to create.

Is that really so much to ask?

Actually, relative to other purchases, businesses demand very similar levels of quality control every day.

We Need a Health Care Package—and a Vendor to Sell It

This entire market model needs to be carefully designed. It will not spring into existence by having anyone micromanaging stand-alone bits and pieces of the current nonsystematic and highly complex infrastructure for either care delivery or care financing in this country.

The new market model needs to be coordinated as a package, not set up as a loose assortment of completely unconnected and disparate pieces—and, as noted above, that entire package needs to be assembled by an infrastructure vendor, purchased by a buyer, and then run effectively by the IV. Each optimal market functionality should be presented by the IV to the buyer as part of a detailed proposal that includes goals, timetables, and operational metrics.

The key for the employers will be to pick the right infrastructure vendors to get the job done. As you can see pretty easily, the

IV role is critically important. Without the existence of the IVs, this market model will not happen. There is a lot of hard work involved, and someone has to actually do it.

The IV needs to be a well-designed entity that sells that entire set of optimal attributes as a package in a viable business model—as a real product. Look at each function that needs to be put in place. Someone needs to be the effective aggregator of all relevant data. Someone needs to track care performance and measure that performance in the context of goals and performance targets. Someone also needs to run the web sites that put needed information about care in the hands of consumers. Someone needs to set up the entire web-based marketplace where consumers can make informed choices about caregivers as well as informed choices about care.

For a market-driven health care marketplace to exist, someone has to put together actual provider networks, help assemble real or virtual care teams, and implement the fundamental elements of interprovider connectivity.

Given American health care's massive care linkage deficiencies, that connectivity will not happen by luck or serendipity. Connectivity needs to be a service provided by someone paid to provide that service in a market environment that both requires and rewards the use of that service. Provider connectivity needs to be embedded in a new market product, defined by specifications and subject to the ongoing expectations of continuous process improvement.

For that total new market context to exist, buyers need to be very clear about the entire product, and then buyers need to pay someone to function as the IV to put that product in place. So can that all be done? I think it can.

The pieces needed for that marketplace exist now to an extent that they did not exist previously. Chapter Five of this book details the new tools that are now available that did not exist before. The single provider number, common electronic claims filing standards, a high level of electronic data flow relative to claims information, and the imminent emergence of areawide electronic health care databases are all tools needed to bring the new consumer-focused market model to full fruition.[2]

Putting that package together needs to be the work of a highly competent vendor—a well-run business unit that sells infrastructure management and reform as a product. That's what makes this proposal and book relatively unique—it assumes that *reform* needs to become a product—a service, assembled and sold by organizations with the skill set, tools, and organizational capacity to do the work. The new array of health industry data tools outlined in previous chapters needs to be used very well by skilled market infrastructure vendors who are hired to make the new market real.

What About Using a "Farmers' Market" or "Connector" Instead of Infrastructure Vendors?

A number of concepts have been offered as potential approaches for how a new health care marketplace based on multiple buyers and sellers (as opposed to single-payer or nationalized health care plans) might be constructed.

Some people believe the market model that could best and most quickly achieve many of those goals is a neutral exchange—a pure "connector" or facilitator, like the stock exchange or mercantile exchange. Such an exchange would be a mechanism for allowing various health plans and health care providers to sell their services in a kind of farmers' market for health coverage and care. In that type of exchange marketplace, multiple health plans and carriers could offer products, and employers could simply give their employees vouchers to use in picking their own health plan. Health plans would, in that model, compete with each other for members and patients.

That exchange type of market could in fact be set up, but it would not create or guarantee care system delivery reform because it could all too easily end up as an exchange for simply purchasing insurance, not care. Insurance competition is good—but care system competition is far better. We need dueling care teams, not dueling underwriters. Real reform of care delivery at core levels will require caregiver competition, not just market battles between insurance actuaries.

To create caregiver retail competition, we need to create care wholesalers—the IVs—the health care megastores who can apply market pressure and offer market incentives to caregivers to institute the needed reforms. In this fully fleshed out marketplace, dueling care teams would compete for the patient dollars. The IVs would set up the context for the competition.

It may be possible and desirable to set up a macro exchange, used for dueling IVs—and that also would be a step forward. But it might be a real challenge to administer. My long-term experience tells me that any mechanism with too many moving parts has a high probability of failure. Elegance in design is often the key to success in performance.

Multiple Vendors and Multiple Markets

We need IVs—but how many do we need? Ideally, in each geographic market, there would be a number of viable infrastructure vendors competing for the role of setting up workable market infrastructures for the buyers. Competition is good. At this stage of the game, I believe it would be premature and strategically shortsighted to build only one market infrastructure per community. Monopolies are generally not an optimal market model for purchasers.

It's also too early in the process to design the ultimately perfect IV. This is the point in the history and development of an exciting and revolutionary new product where creativity should abound—and buyers will be well served if several different vendors come forward, each with its own innovative and highly competitive versions of consumer choice web sites, care management approaches and programs, and insurance coverage benefit designs. It's a time of learning and experimentation, and that learning should be both encouraged by buyers and then directly and immediately subjected to the rigors of toe-to-toe marketplace competition.

Sample Bid Specifications

Buyers need to put in place a bidding process that allows various credible entities to bid for the role of infrastructure reform vendors. The buyers should tell their potential infrastructure vendors that they want each vendor to create a direct and effective marketplace for patients—with one set of market components recognizing, rewarding, and incenting individual provider performance on a defined array of individual provider quality measurements (like the five-year survival rate for breast cancer patients) and the other set of components recognizing, rewarding, structuring, supporting, and guiding caregiver team behaviors in the area of population health, with goals (like cutting second heart attacks by 40 percent or cutting asthma crisis for kids by 75 percent). See Box 7.1 for a sample set of high-level specifications.

Fully Resourced Web Site

The specifications set up by the buyers should require each potential IV to provide a fully resourced web site for patients that facilitates patient choice of caregivers and care approaches. The web site should be tied to each patient's electronic personal health record, and it should feature a care management support system for patients to use for follow-up care support and information, both for acute and chronic diseases.

Consumers are ready to go to the web in increasing numbers for useful information about their care. Ten million of them do every day.[3] The infrastructure vendor for the employer should make that whole communication process very easy, extremely useful, and strategically linked to the IV's overall health improvement agenda.

Box 7.1. Key Points for Infrastructure Vendors: Piecework and Teamwork as Financing Options

1. Incentives for patients and care providers should always focus on and influence the specific behaviors we want to encourage or discourage. Begin with the clear goal—then design the incentive to achieve that goal.

2. *Acute care* is legitimately delivered in incidents of care—and can be paid for and incented as "piecework" with fees for each unit of care.

3. *Chronic care* is best delivered by multiple providers, takes place over time, and is best organized and reimbursed as "teamwork."

4. Piecework and teamwork are best incented with slightly different economic models.

   - Benefit design for piecework should have a base benefit level for each piece of care that requires patients to pay more if they chose to use more expensive providers. Price competition will result.

   - Benefit design for teamwork should have a benefit that incents patients to work with care-registry-supported providers to receive full benefits—and a payment approach that incents or requires team behaviors by caregivers in order for the providers to receive full payment.

5. Both piecework and teamwork should create transparent and accountable data flows—for patients, caregivers, and buyers—about both cost and performance.

Connectivity Between Caregivers

Connectivity between caregivers needs to be an IV assignment, skill set, and agenda. The IV should provide convenient electronic access for all care providers to PHR-level data about each patient—so a specialist treating a particular enrolled patient can go to the IV web site and quickly pull up relevant and needed data about the other care that has been received by that patient from other caregivers. In the case of patients with comorbidities, the IV should have support processes in place to make sure that each of the caregivers involved is aware of the comorbidities and of the care being delivered by the other caregivers. Tools can be created to support that process. Patients need to agree with the data sharing before that work can be done, but I suspect patients will be delighted to get that help. The IVs can use both the web and nurse call lines to support those linkage processes.

Connectivity Between Pharmacists

The IV care information PHR web site for each patient is foundational to these processes. The PHR data set should show prescriptions written, diagnoses made, procedures done, and the general progression of care for each patient. Ideally, that web site should be linked by the IV to a pharmacy program linked to each pharmacy. That program can sort through each patient's prescriptions and send a red flag up when patients receive a prescription that might interact badly with another prescription for that patient. That problem happens relatively often for patients with comorbidities. Each individual specialty practitioner does not always have that data about other prescriptions available. So the IV should take that entire data screening task on as part of the overall IV role. It can be coordinated through the allied pharmacy vendors. This is not an insignificant opportunity to improve care.

The positive impact from that single pharmacy-based functionality could be huge. In one pilot case set up by General Motors, 600,000 prescriptions written by local doctors were run through a computer program that checked for possible dangerous drug interactions. More than 110,000 potential problems were identified in a single year. Nearly 10,000 prescriptions were flagged for creating potential allergy problems for the patients.[4] This is the kind of patient care improvement problem that an IV organization can and should be expected to deal with as part of a new buyer expectation about better linked care.

Certain types of care improvement approaches are relatively easy to do if they are done in the context of an in-place vertically integrated multispecialty provider group like Kaiser Permanente or the Mayo Clinic using an automated medical record system to support each caregiver. In those caregiver team settings, care linkages are expected, and shared data flow is simply the way things work. It's both a cultural and an operational expectation.

But in an environment of unconnected, unlinked, sometimes competing solo practice providers, in far too many cases those kinds of data flow linkages will not simply happen if the solo providers somehow need to create, implement, and maintain the linkages on their own. Why? Because those solo caregivers do not have the tools or the logistical support to make those linkages a consistent reality. Remember the example above. In just one city in just one year, 110,000 drug errors resulted. It took a new computer model to spot these 110,000 potential problem prescriptions. They would not have been detected without that system until the patient was damaged. The best-intentioned individual doctors didn't know those 110,000 potential problems existed. That unlinked and uncoordinated care is not good enough. In the new market model, the IV should be paid to create and sustain those interprovider linkages and to provide that support. It's part of the infrastructure vendor functionality that needs to be built into the buyer's specifications.

Buyer Risk Pool

The infrastructure vendor should also be held accountable by the buyer for creating a detailed database about each buyer's own risk pool, with actuarial and financial information about the employees, family members, and possible retirees covered by the employer. That database should, for starters, profile the overall cost impact and current care performance levels relative to each of the five chronic diseases, along with a detailed plan to improve care delivery and outcomes relative to each disease.

Again, solo providers and hospitals with no contractually linked physicians will not be able to set up needed overall programs for population health improvement on their own. They need help. The IV needs to provide that help. If we want that highly targeted and operationally linked health improvement job done, it needs to be done either directly by a large multispecialty group practice (like Kaiser Permanente, Mayo Clinic, HealthPartners, Intermountain Healthcare, and others) or indirectly through a network of independent caregivers held together in a virtual integration model set up by the various IVs to allow independent caregivers to function in many respects like a Kaiser Permanente or HealthPartners care team. The virtual integration model set up by each IV should be clearly designed, clearly explained, and clearly accountable. Care registries can be an extremely useful care improvement tool for specific diseases like diabetes or asthma. It can be almost impossible to manage chronic care really well without that tool. The IVs should help providers, solo and group, in their networks set up, support, and use those registries, fed initially in most cases by PHR data. Registries are needed. Someone needs to help unlinked providers set them up and use them. IVs can do that job.

How Will Infrastructure Vendors and Core Providers Be Paid?

So how should each infrastructure vendor be paid? Those are particularly important issues to resolve, because the payment model obviously sets up the economic incentive infrastructure for the entire marketplace, caregivers and patients alike. It also will tell us whether any of the businesses currently serving the health care industry would be well suited to reconstitute themselves as IVs.

Cash flow will determine the success or failure of this proposed market model. That cash starts in the hands of the employer—the large buyer—and then gets distributed through two channels to the actual providers of care. The first channel is through the infrastructure vendors. How the IVs get paid will determine what they do. The second channel is the employee-patient. Employers subsidize employee benefit plans. The nature of that subsidy needs to be understood and strategically structured. The benefit design itself also needs to be a tool aimed at achieving the overall objective of market reform. We could simply decide not to make changes in any of those cash flows—continuing to use fee-for-service payments, self-insuring the risk at the employer level, and insulating employees from basic cost and value issues relative to care. That would not create an optimal care reform result.

A cost-plus arrangement built on top of a simple and pure fee-for-service care purchasing model would be easy to implement and easy to account for. However, it would obviously run the risk of perpetuating the classic perverse incentives of the fee-for-service economics that have allowed and encouraged this country to build a massively expensive, uncoordinated, and unlinked care infrastructure supported entirely by a vast and rich river of fees.

That perversely incented fee-for-service payment model has typically been dysfunctionally linked through the design of insurance benefit packages to an economically challenged and problematic insulation of many patients from the actual costs of care. And the total badly structured and badly incented package of employee coverage has typically been funded in its entirety by a premium-linked employer contribution level that perversely masks the growing costs of care. In other words, the benefit packages have typically insulated well-insured patients from any direct incentives relative to care costs. Likewise, the cost-based employer premium subsidies have insulated patients from the need to reduce the overall costs of care or purchase more efficient health plan alternatives. Better decisions could and should be made in both of those categories of funding if we really want to reform care.

Let's start by looking at the cash flow that subsidizes employee benefits. Is our current approach optimal if we want the health care marketplace to be value-based? What alternatives exist? Is there a better way for employers to fund premiums?

An alternative approach to funding health care that a lot of employers are now considering would use more of a "fixed contribution" payment arrangement. In that model, the employer makes a defined and fixed contribution each month to each employee's health care coverage funding, and the employee then makes choices about what set of benefits, coverage options, or health plans he or she wants to purchase with those dollars. If the employees purchase the most expensive health plan or benefits package, the employee pays the additional cost out of their own pocket. Likewise, if an employee selects a health plan whose rates go up faster than other plans, the employee pays those additional costs as well.

Why would that change add any value in the effort to create a well-functioning health care marketplace in America? Because when the employer simply pays for all premium increases and the employee is insulated from those costs, then employees are less likely to favor, appreciate, or select strategies and approaches that reward value and keep premiums at lower levels.

Employee choices in the new context of having a fixed amount of money to spend on health care would obviously create increased employee focus on the cost of various benefit and coverage options. So employees would have an incentive to buy coverage in a competitive, data-rich market model set up by IV vendors who would work hard to keep the overall costs of coverage down.

That is why there could be a benefit for reform in giving employees a fixed amount of money to spend for health care coverage. As my father used to say, people seldom appreciate a solution until they have clearly perceived a problem. Solutions that solve unperceived problems tend not to be supported. So the full array of health care cost solutions stands a higher chance of losing or not earning public and patient approval until there's a sense that those solutions actually help with a problem. In this case, the problem would be that employees would have a fixed amount of money to spend.

We also need to improve benefit design if we are going to more effectively involve patients in the cost and value of care. Current benefit packages tend to be fairly basic in their design, with little or no cost sharing for patients as part of the benefit approach. A far better approach would be to design the benefits to encourage use of the new marketplace to select the best value providers and to encourage effective participation in population health initiatives. Some specific thoughts on these points are shown below.

Let's assume the IV has done its job of designing benefits well. In a new and reformed marketplace with provider performance data available to each consumer, a combination of consumer price sensitivity about the overall purchasing package and patient sensitivity about provider performance at the level of care would set up a very different market dynamic than the one we have now. A marketplace for care would exist, and employees would have both an economic interest in the cost of care and a very personal interest in the quality of care.

From the employer's perspective, the defined contribution cost for health care benefits could be a budgetable decision each year—with a preset, budgetable, fixed contribution number defining and limiting annual employer expense rather than having the expense for each year driven by whatever turns out to be the subsequent cost of the actual benefits that are guaranteed.

To make that approach work for the employees, the care delivery options available from the market model would need to have their own obvious and understandable cost containment dynamics. Employees would be incented to select cost-effective caregivers and caregiver teams if the selection of those teams made the actual coverage options selected by the employee more affordable. Alain Enthoven has spoken at great length on the desirability of this kind of competition between health systems. A fixed contribution approach would also give the infrastructure vendor a major incentive and tool to use to achieve real overall cost savings in order to keep their available premium levels competitive in each relevant marketplace. There is a major opportunity at this point to introduce a much more effective and relevant set of patient choices into the marketplace. Those choices include benefit plans and core systems—individual caregivers and individual health agendas. Choices are good—and the IVs need to be set up to facilitate an appropriate array of choices with cost as a relevant decision factor. A defined contribution approach, done well, can help incent better consumer choices. We don't absolutely need a defined contribution payment approach to make this model work, but it can create a financial context that can be useful.

Benefit Designs Need to Create Consumer Competition

Benefit design will be a very important element in market reform. We need to incent positive behaviors with benefit design. We need to incent proactive care and healthy choices. We need to incent use of the most cost-effective providers. Conversely, it will be important not to place financial barriers in the way for people with chronic conditions who need to do the kinds of proactive things outlined in Chapter Four to forestall and hopefully prevent the debilitating and expensive complications that can arise from their chronic conditions. It will be important to use careful and strategic benefit design to encourage provider price competition and increase the use of cost-efficient care providers. In fact, real price competition between some categories of providers will not exist in any settings until benefit designs change.

Again, the logic is pretty basic. Follow the money. Price competition will not exist between caregivers unless price differences between providers directly affect patient purchasing decisions. It is a very simple concept. Benefit design needs to foster price competition, not stifle it. In far too many cases, the current benefit design works directly against price competition, rather than for it. When the patient copay for all office visits is a flat $20 per visit, why would a provider who now charges $100 a visit ever drop that fee to compete with a provider across the street who charges only $80 a visit? That price drop obviously would not happen. Why? Because the provider would not gain in any way from dropping the price. The provider across the street could cut his or her fee to $70, but the patient would still pay only the exact same $20 copay. The perfectly flat copay benefit approach makes the actual price difference on office visits between any two providers irrelevant. If anything, the accountants and business managers for the lower-price provider should be wondering why they don't charge $100 for their own office visit, just like their competitor.

Let me offer a piece of advice at this point. The next several pages offer some fairly specific thoughts about how to use benefit design to increase price competition between providers. If that topic is not of interest to you, I recommend jumping ahead a few pages to the section How Health Premiums Are Calculated. Everyone should, I believe, understand that point.

Flat Deductible

So what benefit design changes could introduce real provider price competition? A flat deductible can have that effect for some types of care. If everyone had a $1,000 deductible, and each patient had to pay the full cost of each office visit until the $1,000 was spent, then the difference between $70 and $100 would obviously be relevant—at least for initial visits. That $30 per visit additional expense might then cause some patients to select the $70 doctor instead of the $100 doctor.

As deductible plans become more common, we can expect additional patient price sensitivity relative to the categories of care and services that usually fall under the deductible amount. If everyone in America had a $1,000 deductible plan, one result would be that office visit prices would be more visible and real cost competition would likely emerge for some basic, front-end categories of care. However, there is also a serious strategic downside to simply using flat deductibles, as we saw in Chapter Three. Flat deductibles tend to discourage chronic disease patients from getting needed preventive and maintenance care. A stand-alone flat deductible can encourage cost sensitivity at the expense of overall care expenses. So a flat deductible could create very desirable price competition for certain levels of care, but the people who spend 75 percent of our care dollars (chronic care patients) would not receive the services and drugs they need to reduce the total costs of their care.

Flat Percentage

Another benefit approach that might work to increase cost sensitivity by patients in some cases is to ask patients to cover and pay a flat percentage of every bill. The flat percentage approach would, of course, result in patients paying a bit more money if they use a higher-priced caregiver. It's just arithmetic. If the patient pays 20 percent of each bill, then the patient will pay more if the caregiver fee is higher and less if the fee is lower. In a 20 percent copay arrangement, a patient would pay $16 for an $80 physician visit and $20 for a $100 office visit. That four dollars is, of course, a cost difference.

The problem is it's really not much of a difference. Under that plan, only 20 percent of any fee difference would be seen or felt by the patient. Eighty percent of the provider price difference would still be masked by the benefit plan. That's just how the math works. So would patients actually change doctors to save only 20 percent of any difference in unit provider charges? They might if the issue involves a $1,000 procedure versus an $800 procedure. But probably not for a few dollars' difference in office visit fees.

It's also very important to remember that a pure deductible might create direct competition relative to primary care fees, but even a large deductible would be completely irrelevant to incent or influence any price-based choices when provider prices for any given service exceed the deductible. A flat percentage copayment, on the other hand, would be relevant for very expensive care items, but not very effective relative to less costly units of care.

Community Competition Fee Alignment

A more direct way to create a price leverage decision point for the consumer would be to base the actual benefit paid for each service on a lower price charged for that exact same particular service in a given community. That approach would create a very direct price competition impact because the lowest price in each market would set the benefit level for that service for each market. So under that approach if there is an $80 office visit price at one clinic and $100 at another, the benefit payment made by the coverage plan for all patients at either clinic would be $80–the lower local price for that service. Any patient who went to a higher-priced provider would have to pay the cost difference between the two fees. A patient who used the $100 provider, in other words, would simply pay the $20 price difference. All of it. Out of his or her pocket.

That's actually very direct price competition. It invokes pure market forces. In that case, if the payment rule is that the lowest-priced credible local provider actually determines the base payment for the local benefit package, then the price charged by the lowest cost provider in each area would have extreme and absolutely direct market relevance, and the higher-priced providers would have an equally direct market incentive to bring down their prices.

It's an interesting concept. Market forces would be fully engaged. Providers could still choose to ignore the pricing decisions made by a key competitor, but they would now face the market consequences. Also, any decision by a given provider to charge more money than the base fee for the same service in a market would not cause the overall price of premiums paid by the employer to be higher. Why? Because the cost to the employer as the payer for that service would drop to the lowest local market price. The claims for both providers would be paid at the same low price. Any patient who chose the more expensive provider would pay the price difference out of pocket.

From the perspective of pure market economics, that community-based fee adjustment benefit approach is almost a perfect payment model. It introduces direct price competition between providers of care, but maintains full coverage for the patients who decide to get their care from the lower-priced local caregiver. Consumers who want to "buy up" to a higher-priced provider or care site could do that freely. But their decision to use higher-priced (but not higher-quality) care would affect only them. Their decision to use a more expensive provider would not raise the premiums for the other patients in their insurance pool. Given the existence of nine thousand billing codes for care, the real-world application of this approach should be limited to a subset of high-leverage, high-volume, potentially price-competitive services. Basic office visits are one good example of a service that could be encouraged to be price-competitive. Obstetric (OB) packages are another. OB groups could offer other prices for a complete prenatal-through-delivery care package. Those prices now vary hugely. Price competition might be useful. Each IV should work with the buyer to figure out which conditions should be paid for in this way. In most settings, that competitive pricing approach could be used for a select but significant number of care-related prices and procedures, including orthopedic surgery, OB care, general office visits, and later extended to a wider range of other somewhat discretionary, nonemergency categories of care. The Internet is essential to this market model. Without the Internet, it would be impossible for the IVs to identify which services are subject to price competition and which prices are relevant to the patient-consumer. This model would not work with a paper-based system.

The danger of that pricing approach would be that every local provider might base her prices on the prices of every other provider—so no one has any price advantage or disadvantage. In every market, it will take at least one significant provider eager for patient volume to set each local base price. In a lot of settings, that will happen. In some, it will not, and then it will be the job of the infrastructure vendor and maybe the buyers as a coalition to inspire at least one key provider to be a cost leader. In markets with no price competition, the buyer and IV may simply choose a "fair" price derived from other markets and use that price to set the local price tone. Wal-Mart, Best Buy, and Target create a very similar model for TV sets by making sure their customers always have a set of low-cost television choices.

If no competition occurs, then a very similar market dynamic can be created by having the IV simply assign a "fair" price as the base price for a given service in a given area. Buyers would need to support that decision if and when employees expressed unhappiness about that benefit level.

Base Prices Can Be Assigned or Bid

The best way to get this started would be for the IVs in each market to select which local procedures ought to be subjected to the new base price market competition model. Buyers need to be partners in developing these lists. This whole approach would need to be very clearly communicated both to all patients and to all local providers. Paper, as noted earlier, will not get that job done. But it could be fairly easily administered on the web. In fact, without the web, it would be an impossible benefit concept to administer. Basing benefits on the low-cost provider definitely would introduce price competition to selected areas of care. It would function very much like the role of a Target, Wal-Mart, or Best Buy in getting vendors to offer at least one set of very competitive products to their retail customers.

For some categories of care, of course, price competition will not or cannot affect patient decision making. It's impossible—or at least extremely impractical—to price shop for cardiologists in the middle of a heart attack. I can confirm that from recent experience. As I noted earlier, I currently have time to write this book because I recently had a heart attack followed by heart bypass surgery. I can tell you absolutely that I was in no position to check out competitive prices for cardiology, or even hospital room rates, in the middle of my attack. Had I been pregnant, however, it would have been possible to price shop for both obstetricians and a delivery room in the time prior to giving birth. And if one OB group in town charged $4,000 for prenatal care and a normal delivery, and another equally qualified group charged $6,000, I believe those price differences would affect my judgment about OB groups very directly—but only if I had to pay the actual cost difference out of my own pocket.

For units of care where the IVs determine that pure price competition is not the best mechanism, a major role for the IV needs to be to negotiate the very best prices with care providers. IVs need to do volume purchasing to get best prices for some services (lab tests, for example) and set up price competition to incent best prices for other services. Benefit designs need to be set up so the actual and relevant lab tests can be effectively, safely and functionally channeled to the lowest bidder.

Pricing in Vertically Integrated Plans

In my own case with my heart attack, prices were not at all relevant. I knew exactly what hospital to go to. I had pretty complete coverage, and I used health plan providers for care, so unit price differences between hospitals were completely irrelevant to me anyway. My own health plan already had a very good price set up with the hospital I was in. That price was part of the premium charged by my health plan to my employer for my coverage.

In the new market model, for consumers who elect to receive their care from an integrated team of caregivers, those kinds of individual care unit prices would still not be relevant, because each price would be part of the total premium paid to the total care team. Someone needs to be very price-sensitive. In the case of vertical integration, the price sensitivity is embedded in the total process. But for those patients who choose nonintegrated, virtually integrated or purely nonsystem approaches to care, unit prices can and should be very relevant, and the benefit package needs to support that relevance.

For nonsystems of care, if we really want to see providers compete on price, then the benefit package of the future can and should be redesigned to include price-related benefits for certain categories of care. As I noted, a really effective model could base the competition for certain units and categories of care on the best price charged by credible local providers of care.

The Importance of Price Competition

Price competition is needed to bring care costs down. Price competition does not happen now at the unit of care level, and that competition will not happen unless prices for each unit are very directly relevant. Ideally, price competition should take place both for units of care and for aggregated health care premiums. As Alain Enthoven said clearly two decades ago, in a 401(k)-like health care financing model with fixed employer contributions, the premiums charged for each benefit plan would be extremely and directly relevant to each covered person. When the health coverage payment from the employer simply covers the full premium of whatever plan the employee chooses, then the variable premium numbers for each health plan are obviously less relevant. All prices would be paid. But if the fixed contribution paid by the employer is based on the premiums charged by the lowest-cost coverage vendor, and if employees pay the difference between that low-cost vendor and the higher-cost plans out of their own pocket, then any plans offered by the buyer would each have a direct incentive to have the lowest price. That particular fixed-level payment approach creates price competition between plans.

How Health Premiums Are Calculated

Understanding how health coverage premiums are calculated is a good thing at this point in the discussion.

In other forms of insurance—life insurance, disability insurance, fire and accident insurance, and so forth—the actuarial formulas used to set prices can be pretty complicated. The people doing the math to calculate the rate for those forms of insurance have to estimate multiyear issues like changing life expectancy, likely future interest rates, the projected cost of money in every relevant future year, and even scientific guesses on topics like whether or not hurricanes are on the upswing. Setting premium rates for those kinds of insurance is really hard.

Care Drives Cost

Health coverage rating is pretty simple. And immediate. The prices for premiums are typically not calculated a decade or more in advance. They are incredibly immediate. The premium price is simply set this year for next year. How are they set? Using addition and long division. It's pretty basic. For major buyers, the ultimate cost of the per-employee premium is just the cost of all claims paid this year divided by the number of people covered. For small groups and individuals, all expenses for people in your category are pooled and the premiums are calculated based on the total cost of the pool. That total cost of claims paid is the expense. An average claims expense for each member is calculated by adding up the total cost of claims and then dividing the total cost of care by the total number of covered members. That number becomes the base rate. Then actuaries try to guess how much more expensive claims will be for that group of people for next year. That estimate is a premium inflation factor. This year's average cost is multiplied by that inflation number. The rating people then add on a flat administrative cost, add in taxes if any are relevant, and then add a target margin or profit for the insurer, and that's the rate people get charged.[5]

The margin and administrative cost tend to be pretty flat year over year as a percentage of premiums. So the absolute driver of 85 percent to 90 percent of all premium costs each year is the direct, actual, and immediate cost of care—and that number is calculated by adding up the total number of claims paid in the prior year for the covered population.

Where do those claims costs come from? As we discussed earlier, claims are the bills that the providers send to the payer for the services provided to patients. Providers include doctors, hospitals, pharmacies, labs, imaging centers, and so forth. Those costs are all added together. It's just arithmetic. If the cost of the pharmacy goes up 20 percent in a year, that claims payment number goes into the claims total. The new average cost of care is then calculated, and the premium directly increases as a result of drug prices going up. Likewise, if hospital costs go up, premiums go up. If medical costs go up, premiums go up. It's a very simple model. For large group plans, premium is driven directly by the costs of care for their employees. For small groups and individuals, the premiums are based on the total cost of claims for all small groups and individuals in their cost pool.

Competition Will Cut Costs

The lesson from that basic exercise in arithmetic is that to reduce premiums, the strategy has to be to somehow reduce the costs of care as measured by the cost of claims. So how do we bring the costs of care down? That's the key question. Improving care for the 1 percent of the population who incur 35 percent of our claims costs would help a lot. If their claims went down by 10 percent, that number would cut the premium costs by 3.5 percent.

The very best way of reducing health care premiums is by improving the care given to the people with chronic conditions who incur 75 percent of our total care costs—to the point where the costs of care for that population shrink by 10 percent, 20 percent, or more. Simply bringing those costs to a flat position would end major premium cost increases. For the various unit costs of care and for various care levels that involve acute care versus chronic care, the benefit changes I mentioned earlier could be useful. The benefit approach I mentioned earlier that sets actual benefit levels in a community based on the prices charged by the local lowest-cost provider of care would very likely cut both the costs of care and the cost of premiums charged. If a local infrastructure vendor reached out to all of the providers in their city to negotiate office visit prices, and the lowest credible price was $80, then that $80 could be what every future office visit claim would cost the payer. The $100 visits and $120 visits charged by other providers would simply shrink to $80 as an actual paid claim benefit, so the total cost of claims paid would go down and the total premium would go down—all other prices being equal. Introducing cost competition in a way that reduces claims costs is one direct route to reducing premium costs. As noted earlier, this approach should be applied to a select set of procedures.

Some skill would definitely be needed to determine what fee level should be used as the base for each benefit in the community. If there are a thousand doctors doing patient visits in a town, and only one solo practice dropped its prices to an $80 fee, it would probably be a bad idea to use that number for that purpose. If all of the providers' bids for a service are too high, the IV should just set the base fee at a "fair" price.

This is a very different approach to benefit design. Employers would need to directly involve their employees in making cost-based care decisions, instead of shielding patients from any real differences in the cost of care. Some patients will be unhappy about paying more for deciding to use a higher-cost provider. Communication about the approach will need to be very well managed.

Patients are more likely to accept that benefit model if the absolutely direct relationship between the costs of claims and the costs of premiums is well understood. That's often not true today. A surprising number of people believe health care premiums are somehow set by health plans arbitrarily, with no direct linkage to costs. I once heard a national journalist say that the number one factor driving up health care costs was the increasing price of premiums. Other than being 180 degrees wrong and completely reversing the actual real-world-cost causality, that was a fascinating insight into how quite a few people think.

Many care providers will hate the competitive fee pricing model. Games will be played. And fairness needs to be built into the pricing approach. If one hospital in town charges $10,000 for a normal medical stay for a given condition and the next hospital down the street charges $20,000 for that exact same stay, should the entire difference be paid by the patient?

Some judgment is needed. It may make sense to phase in a price difference of that magnitude over time, with patients amply forewarned. But conversely, if we don't in some way reflect in our patient choices and benefit packages the fact that one hospital in town has chosen to charge twice as much for exactly the same care, then we will never remedy the price piece of the health care cost dilemma.

Keep in mind what is possible. Price competition in health care can happen.

Laser Surgery Example

Look at laser surgery for eyes as an example of what happens when pure price competition is introduced into the delivery of care. Lasers are now used in eye surgery to correct nearsightedness. That is not a benefit covered by insurance, so patients have had to pay out of pocket for that eye care over the past decade or so since the procedure was invented. What happened when prices for that particular surgery were subject to the rigors of direct price competition?

Five years ago, that surgery cost $2,200 per eye.[6] With competition, the price dropped to $1,500 per eye, $1,000 per eye, $500 per eye—and in some very aggressive settings I've seen the surgery marketed as low as $300 per eye—roughly one eighth of the original price. It's not clear if those advertised prices represent all costs for each patient, but there is no doubt that the prices dropped dramatically.

Along the way, for many practitioners, the quality of the surgery improved. So, in essence, we now have better surgery for slightly over a tenth of the cost. What happened? Price competition and market forces worked. The entire process of laser eye surgery was completely reengineered. The equipment was reengineered, the support staff was reengineered, the painkillers were reengineered. The surgeons now move their equipment from patient to patient rather than moving the patients to the equipment, which means they no longer have to wait until the next patient is ready. A surgeon can now perform numerous surgeries a day.[7]

I talked to a senior executive for one of the companies that made one version of the laser surgery equipment. He said they repeatedly reengineered that equipment top to bottom, cutting cost and improving effectiveness. The equipment is now stainless steel, not painted. The number of bolts needed to build it was reduced. The equipment moves far better. And faster.

Everything happened that should have happened in any good reengineering process. It looked a lot like the kinds of reengineering that took $300 DVD players and turned them into better quality DVD players a decade later for under $50. Reengineering works.

Opportunities to Reengineer

So what would happen to office visits if that whole area of health care suddenly become directly price competitive? Would any waiting rooms be reengineered? Would the role of nurses change? Would anything in the room design or patient check-in process become more effective or efficient?

Would e-visits substitute for more expensive office visits at a fraction of the cost? Would people figure out how to provide and sell some categories of basic care delivery functions and patient visits in discount stores or pharmacies?

Once that total care reengineering process got underway, the possibilities would be endless. Care could be better and less expensive, with caregivers using computers more effectively both as care support tools and as patient support tools. Remember the question earlier about why computers haven't helped cut costs in health care. If we had a competitively priced market for primary care, does anyone believe computers would not find themselves used in the same efficiency-enhancing ways they are used in other industries?

Likewise, if the goal is to cut congestive heart failure admissions in half, does anyone believe that the whole computerized patient health record database—and condition-specific, strategically implemented computerized care registries—would not be main tools to get that job done? We are on the cusp of an increased level of computer support for health care that will spring from health care finally having an incentive to perform well in a number of areas where computers could actively and effectively provide support.

Infrastructure Vendors Can Improve Data Flow

As I noted earlier, the massive data deficit of American health care needs to be alleviated somewhat in order for caregivers to systematically improve care. When the combined electronic database of all claims-paying organizations is available to the infrastructure vendors in an integrated form for tracking overall provider performance and for figuring out how well a community is doing relative to important issues like asthma care and congestive heart failure interventions—and when that same database facilitates tracking of individual provider performance in key areas like five-year post-surgery survival rates for breast cancer patients—then setting goals for improved care and channeling patients to the right providers will also be possible. If the benefits are well designed to both support preventive and maintenance care and encourage direct price competition between providers, then those elements of an effective marketplace will also come into play.

Do not underestimate the potential usefulness of the PHR as a tool for doctors to use in taking care of patients. Buyers need to insist that their infrastructure vendors make full use of those tools. The very best model for coordinated patient care is still a fully integrated physician group and care system using a shared electronic medical record. But progress can be made in other settings.

Use Personal Health Records to Create Virtual Integration

The logistical advantages of a single team of physicians working with both shared and complete patient data are fairly obvious. But for those practitioners who do not already function in a group and who specialize by disease category, one care-related goal for the IVs needs to be to help the nonsystem caregivers to create the functional benefits of being in a "virtual group"—to create a set of connectivity mechanisms and data flow tools that let each specialist taking care of a patient know what the other providers who are treating that same patient are discovering and doing.

Buyers should demand that their infrastructure vendor make electronic tools available to support that process. It's a reasonable request and it's really the only viable way for today's unlinked independent providers of care to facilitate improved linkages with any consistency. Doctors need easy access to that information. They need to be able to pull down from the web a relevant set of claims-based information about each patient. That same IV-run data flow process should warn doctors about potentially problematic drug interactions. And it should generate a reminder to caregivers, care managers, and patients when certain levels of needed care are or are not being delivered.

Infrastructure Vendors Will Use Personal Health Records to Prevent Care Linkage Deficiencies

Remember the patient support needs described in Chapter Two. At a very simple level, if a diabetic patient has gone for a dangerously long time without having his or her eye damage levels checked, then the IV's computer should send a reminder to the patient, and a reminder should appear on the computer of whatever caregiver the patient has selected for treating his diabetes. It should also appear on the computers of other caregivers taking care of that patient for other conditions.

Similarly, the IV's integrated computer database program should check to see that each child has all immunizations and should remind both parents and, where known, the child's primary caregivers that specific immunizations seem to be needed. When that child shows up in any doctor's office for care, that doctor should be able to go to the infrastructure vendor's web site to get a claims-based profile on that child, and the profile should contain a prompt saying, "These immunizations are not currently on file." The specific messages will need to evolve within each IV and within each medical specialty area, but they do need to exist and be used.

Disease Registries

It's obviously very possible to manage care better with electronic tools that fall short of a full electronic medical record (EMR). Disease registries are one example. As discussed in Chapter Two, a disease registry is a computerized program designed to keep track of care issues for people with a specific disease. For example, a disease registry for diabetes will track medications, eye exams, blood sugar levels, and so forth—all needed types of care for people with diabetes. Doctors consult the registry when they provide care for the patient, tracking care over time to make sure it conforms to best practice.

Disease registries can be a wonderful, highly focused tool that reminds caregivers electronically of needed care for a specific and targeted subset of patients. Until IVs can implement a fully functional, interactive EMR database, they should be required to support such disease registries. Registries can be triggered by claims-based data and then set up on computers to provide additional clinical data and care follow-up for selected patients.

Such disease registries are being used to good effect now, even without the benefit of aggregated claim-based databases. Denver Health, for example, has created computerized disease registries that keep track of selected care issues for patients with a couple of chronic conditions. The computerized registries remind the caregivers of what care those patients need. Information is updated at every patient visit. The results have been extremely positive, with a significant drop in disease complications and a major increase in science-based, medical best practice protocol compliance.

Buyers should require the IVs they hire to support registries where providers create them by feeding them with timely claims-based data. The IVs should also facilitate and support the creation of those registries with local teams of caregivers. Benefit design could require both providers and patients with specific conditions to utilize the registries in order to receive full benefits.

There is a lot of low-hanging fruit to be harvested in these areas. It's not possible to do everything at once. But a lot can be done quickly. The process can start with a focus on the key chronic diseases. Each IV can show each buyer the processes, network configurations, and benefit design approaches that will be used by the infrastructure vendor to have an impact on each disease. Performance needs to be tracked, showing both actual care outcome improvements (heart attack reduction rates) and care process enhancements (web sites that get extensive use in the support of better care).

Infrastructure Vendors Should Support Best Personal Health Practices

A key to the success of the entire care improvement agenda will be to get consumers more involved in maintaining, protecting, and restoring their own health. The potential positive impact of patients giving up cigarettes, losing weight, and exercising regularly are massive, actually exceeding anything we can achieve in the short term by improving care delivery. The ideal outcome for health care reform in America would be to have nonsmoking, low-weight, physically active people receiving their care from an outcomes-based, continuously improving, scientifically current, and extremely efficient care system. The potential dollar impact of achieving all of those goals would allow us to significantly reduce total health care costs in America while covering everyone and taking full advantage of the next generation of technologically advanced diagnostic tools and care delivery approaches. Medicare funding would disappear as an issue if we could achieve those goals. Our ability to benefit from the advances of medical science would also be enhanced significantly if we set up a value-based, data-rich payment model that involves patient cost sharing in the most appropriate ways.

To get to the end point of better patient health behaviors, each infrastructure vendor needs to be required by the buyers to bring extensive health education tools to the table. Culture changes are also possible—and are needed. The care delivery system, working in partnership with employers, needs to help set up a new culture of healthy eating and healthy activity levels. Smoking needs to be discouraged, if not penalized, and people who smoke need to be given support to end their use of nicotine.

Financial Penalties as Incentives

How can patients be incentivized to improve their health? For example, how can smokers be incentivized to quit? One fairly obvious possibility is to use financial penalties. Rather than penalize people at the point of care, where benefit reductions for smokers can have the unintended and undesirable consequences of having patients avoid necessary care, it probably makes more sense to require smokers to pay more in monthly premiums, an approach very similar to raising auto premiums for people with a record of accidents or infractions. Monthly premiums for smokers could be adjusted significantly upward after, for example, a two-year warning period.

Enforcing a penalty via premiums would be very difficult for many obvious reasons, but it might be a useful penalty just for the message it sends. And if it does nothing other than force smokers to hide their smoking for large portions of each day, that act of hiding by itself will probably cut down the total level of smoking for those people. One large employer has gone a step further and uses a Breathalyzer-type device to test whether employees are smoking.[8] Employees have been fired for not taking the test. Other employers are looking at not hiring smokers at all. Simply increasing the monthly premiums for those folks might be a better idea. In any case, times are changing. Health is becoming an imperative in quite a few sites. Health is our greatest opportunity. Improving care by 50 percent for diabetics is wonderful, but not as wonderful as reducing the number of diabetics by 50 percent by preventing the disease.

This book is primarily about health care delivery and financing reform, with a focus on using technology and the marketplace to improve health care costs, efficiency, and quality. It's not about all of the steps we can and should take as a culture to persuade people to more highly value and practice healthy behaviors. Those personal health improvement agendas are incredibly important—and they need to be the topic of another book and a key goal of U.S. health care policy.

Rewarding Healthy Behavior

For now, the recommendation is that each infrastructure vendor be required by the buyer through the specification-setting process to provide an extensive set of health-influencing support tools, ranging from individual health consults to group sessions to computer system–based health education materials to benefit design models that encourage health and possibly penalize certain less healthy behaviors. It's definitely possible to design benefit packages that either reward or penalize certain weight levels. It's also possible to reward or penalize certain aspects of personal health status.

I talked to a businessperson from India recently whose company was planning to increase or decrease the monthly premium charged to people with diabetes by whether or not they were successfully controlling their blood sugar. Using periodic tests, the tentative plan is to double the monthly premium costs for people whose blood sugar levels exceed a defined target level twice in a row. The premium would stay doubled until the blood sugar levels dropped back to target ranges and stayed there for a specified period of time. The company was working on the technology needed to make that monitoring process simple and doable.

Is that whole approach a good line of thought? Should there be a direct financial incentive—either a penalty or a reward—for people with diabetes to manage their own blood sugar? Likewise, should we arrange for someone who is already significantly overweight to be penalized if their personal body mass index score goes up over time? Who would set those goals? What would be a fair measurement? A fair penalty? What approach would not be in effect purely discriminatory in an unfair or illegal way? These are very interesting questions.

Should premium or benefit dollars be linked to personal health decisions and, if so, how should they be fairly and accurately linked? Since health care premiums are simply the total cost of care divided by the total number of covered people, if one person acts in deliberately unhealthy ways, those subsequent costs do in fact make everybody's premiums go up. Is that total cost increase fair to everyone else, particularly to the people who don't smoke, who watch their weight, and who regularly exercise? It's a matter for ethicists as well as economists to ponder. As I said, those are all fascinating topics for another book. For now, the immediate issue is what buyers should do to have the maximum positive impact on the care system itself.

How can we take the massive, uncoordinated, marginally accountable, and excessively expensive infrastructure of American health care delivery and re-align the many wonderful parts of that infrastructure to achieve the kinds of choices and accountability that we need?

That infrastructure reform process will not happen on its own.

As I said earlier, someone needs to be hired to do that job. Hospitals will not spontaneously set up effective pre-asthma prevention programs that will eliminate $10,000 to $20,000 admissions in exchange for no financial reward and no cash flow. Clinics and physicians whose revenue comes from asthma patients needing care can't economically volunteer their time to set up asthma crisis prevention programs for large numbers of patients so that those patients need no care. Those prevention jobs need to be done. They won't happen until somebody does them. That somebody—the IV—needs to be hired. And paid, to make sure the job is done.

Pure Provider Prepayment

There are two payment approaches available to us to get that work done. One is pure provider prepayment. When a group of providers is prepaid as a team to take total care of all patients, including all asthma patients in their patient panel, then the providers have a complete obligation to provide all needed care and a fixed amount of prepaid money to spend to provide that care. Better asthma care costs less money. So well-organized, fully prepaid teams of providers have both the right economic incentive and the right care linkage tools to get that total job done. That is a very good financial model for health care.

But that prepaid, team-based care model with total care accountability will not work for most of American health care. Why? Because two-thirds of providers practice alone.[9] Team-based care strategies are pretty hard to do in solo practice. Also, most solo practitioners do not have complete accountability for the care of any given patient. A patient might go to Doctor A one day for asthma care, but then that very same patient might go to Doctor B another day and Doctor C on a third care encounter a month later. So which of those doctors should or even could be prepaid for that patient's total care? Which of those doctors could be fully accountable for that patient? The answer is, None of them can do the full job.

That's not good. "None" is not a sufficient answer if we want to reform health care.

Obviously, someone needs to be accountable or consistent patient education and systematic care follow-up will not happen. Doctor A will never know whether or not the patient filled his or her prescription, and Doctor B will probably never know whether or not the patient ended up in the emergency room or even in a hospital bed for an asthma crisis. Why won't each doctor know? Because in an unlinked nonsystem of care, no one has the job of sharing that kind of information with and between caregivers. No caregiver even has all of that information. Neither Doctor A, B, or C has the full set of information about each patient. None of those doctors has the tools or wherewithal to get that information, even if they want it. That's just the way it is with the current infrastructure of American health care.

So if we want that job done, it has to be assigned to someone. Telling Doctors A, B, and C to communicate better will not be successful, even if they each try to do that. How could any doctor figure out where each patient of theirs went for their next visit? What would they communicate? Who would they communicate with?

Let me say the obvious truth one more time. If we want that job done, it has to be assigned to someone. Someone has to be hired to do that job. Who should that be? And who in the total world of American health care financing and health care delivery has the right vantage point, sufficient leverage, the logistical wherewithal, and the economic strength and organizational motivation to actually make that assignment?

Buyer Specifications for Infrastructure Vendors

That's where the buyer specifications come into play. Major American buyers need to hire infrastructure vendors to do that work, and the specifications for those IVs need to call explicitly for that full array of work to be done. For this market model to work, the IV hired by the buyer needs, as I noted earlier, to set up computer support systems to track care delivery. The IV needs to make electronic claims-based information about each patient available to each doctor, so Doctor C can tap into that payer database to learn that this patient has seen two prior doctors for his asthma care and that prescriptions were not filled in either case.

The infrastructure vendor also needs to sort through its database to look at all asthma patients to figure out which patients are going to the emergency room and which are not filling their prescriptions. The IV needs to assign case managers—public health nurses, if need be—to each such patient to help the patient navigate the system in order to get best care and avoid future asthma attacks. Or further congestive heart failure attacks.

That work needs to be done. It cannot and will not be done until someone is hired to do it.

Creating Vertically Integrated Care

The role of the new infrastructure vendor needs to be to create, coordinate, and facilitate the functional equivalent of a vertically integrated care system—to create a virtual system that will provide the benefits of coordination, proactive interventions, quality care monitoring, and informed patient choices for each patient. Again, that works needs to be done. It will not happen unless it's assigned to someone who is paid to get it done.

This approach does not turn the solo doctors and the independent hospitals of America magically into integrated caregiving or business units. That task would be far beyond the scope of this strategy. But this approach does move in that direction. It does increase hugely the levels of patient-focused information coordination between those otherwise isolated and independent care units. Someone needs to case manage the congestive heart failure patients. That work is hugely important. Hospitals can't be expected to do that work on their own. They don't have the tools, linkages, or patient contact mechanisms to get that job done. The heavy lifting needs to be done outside of the hospital so that very heavy lifting does not need to be done inside the hospital.

Again, somebody needs to be paid to do that work, or it will not be done. Doing that work well requires systematic thinking, proactive interventions, and focused coordination between caregivers. That's easy work in the context of a true vertically integrated care team, like Kaiser Permanente, HealthPartners, or the Mayo system, but it's work that doesn't happen at all in most other settings. So buyers need to build that work into the specifications for the IVs they hire to get up their benefit delivery approach for their employees.

Vertically Linked Versus Virtually Linked Care

Let me insert a brief description of the value of offering competing system approaches into the discussion at this point. Some care systems—like the one that employs me—already are vertically integrated organizations, with hospitals, physicians, pharmacies, imaging, lab, and related care facilities already all under the same roof. Our parts work well together now. We believe we can do better, but we already do a lot of things well.

We are currently investing billions of dollars in computer systems to enhance care and let us fully realize the full benefits of our in-place structural systemness. We believe that we will be able to use our new multibillion-dollar electronic tool kit to make significant improvements in our care delivery compared to the nonsystems that make up so much of American health care. Our nurses, primary care doctors, specialists, and subspecialists are a team now, and we will be even more of a team when we get all of the systems and process improvement tools we are building in place. We will be particularly effective at helping patients with comorbidities—the relatively small number of people with multiple conditions who truly drive up most health care expenses for us and everyone else.

What we have to offer as a total package will, we believe, help set up a new standard and public expectation for what is actually possible relative to care delivery, effectiveness, and systemness. So why do I mention that issue here? Because in an optimal, performance-based marketplace, we believe it will strengthen the competitive environment to have our entire patient-focused systemness as one of the options consumers can pick as their care and coverage choice. Consumers need choices. Systems and systemness, we believe, should be included in those choices. Real systems and, where those are not available, IV-created virtual systems.

One very important role of the IVs will be to use their array of organizational tools to create computer-linked virtual systems. The virtual systems will be able to compete in selected markets with actual brick-and-mortar physically and functionally organized systems. A number of buyers have wanted us to break up our total package of care at Kaiser Permanente into pieces so the buyers can buy various pieces of our structure separately. We are flattered, but we generally refuse to do that because buying just part of what we do is not the best way to realize our value. We've built our model to be a true package—a linked and integrated package. Our pieces do not work quite as well in a splintered way. Nor do we want to sell disaggregated services. Our strength is team care, so we believe that it is best for the patients and the overall delivery of care when our team is offered to patients as a team.

In the new world this book is advocating—with patients making informed choices about caregivers—it will be a good idea to make us, and other vertically integrated organizations like us, available to members and patients as a package and a team, not just as individual caregivers. We strongly believe the team performance will outperform nonteam performance for quality, value, and cost. The market model needs to have performance data and metrics for all caregivers—including our caregivers—but consumers definitely should be able to select us and organizations like us as a team, and not just as their local nephrologist or urologist. Our doctors practice as a team, achieve as a team, are paid as a team, and it would be counter to the values of the team model we have built to treat our patients in a nonteam context.

So the choices that might exist for individual patients in the new market model could start with patients being able to choose first between receiving care in a vertically integrated approach or from a nonintegrated, virtually linked approach. Other sets of unlinked caregivers will want to use various connectivity tools and data tracking to look like us. The IVs should use these tools wisely to create virtual care systems where physical care systems aren't available. That's a very good thing to do. Virtual systems are in fact what this book is recommending for the rest of the care delivery world that is not vertically integrated. Virtual systems need to be a choice for informed customers. So should real systems. An optimal marketplace should offer both models.

Why should both approaches be offered? In part because it would be immensely ironic if everyone in health care were reorganizing to function in key ways like a vertically integrated organization and then to set up a market dynamic that denies consumers the opportunity to actively choose to get their care from a real vertically integrated organization. It would also be a bit ironic and counterproductive to break up a well-functioning care team into nonlinked pieces at the same time we are trying to get all of the splintered pieces of the rest of American health care to function as a team. We believe patients need health care teams as a choice. When the employees for a given employer make their annual benefit and coverage approach decision, the proposed market choice model in those geographic markets where actual vertically integrated care systems do exist should be to allow employees to chose first between real vertically linked systems and virtual systems. Then, if virtual systems are selected, consumers need to make informed choices between individual caregivers and partial care teams. It will be important to carefully track the results of that competition.

Competition between real systems, virtual systems, and nonsystems in a world where performance data for all caregivers is recorded and transparent will give us a rich array of comparative effectiveness data that will help refine and define the way care will ultimately be delivered in America.

In any case, if employers contract with infrastructure vendors to create an easy-to-use, electronically supported market for care—and if the employees then make choices between various care networks and care delivery approaches based on data about both performance and price, we will be halfway to the new market agenda. The infrastructure vendors will use their creativity, ingenuity, and direct care management experience to both create the new market model and influence the cost of care—in part by targeting both the patients most in need of support and the caregivers most in need of process improvement.

Benefit Delivery Packages

In this new proposed market approach, buyers won't just purchase insurance benefits from IVs—they will purchase benefit delivery packages and a health reform agenda, with multiple layers of accountability within the IV for improving the quality and effectiveness of care. This is a step beyond what buyers have consciously purchased in the past. It will be a significant stretch for many of the organizations that currently sell insurance or coverage administration services to the major employers to extend to selling benefit delivery packages. For some current vendors, it will be a stretch too far—and they will not be able to compete. For other vendors who fully appreciate the changing world of standardized claims data, single provider numbers, electronic claims submission, and the obvious need to improve the accountability and effectiveness of care delivery, this could be a major market opportunity.

The next chapter deals briefly with the possible groups and payers who could take on the role of the IV. There are numerous credible options. Governmental units could decide to try to create local marketplaces, using that newly available set of electronic aggregated claims-based data. Provider organizations or provider coalitions could also decide to bid on the IV business. Buyer coalitions could come together to form their own market infrastructure in some markets. Existing vertically integrated care systems like the Mayo Clinic, Geisinger Clinic, or Kaiser Permanente could step up to take on that role in quite a few markets. Existing health plans could realign their priorities and take on the new IV role. Any and all of those options should be welcomed to the market because both competition and creativity would be increased by having a wider variety of alternative approaches.

Having the government arbitrarily declare itself to be the only available local infrastructure vendor as a care management monopoly would obviously be less than encouraging for both competition and creativity, so it would probably be better not to use that alternative as a key strategy. By contrast, the new role of the government as a major player in feeding previously confidential government program data about care delivery and care costs into the aggregated data set while insuring absolute patient confidentiality and security in the ultimate use of that aggregated data will, for obvious reasons, be highly beneficial to this overall market-based strategic direction for American health care.

What This New Marketplace Will Look Like

So what are the next steps? Buyers need to decide whether or not to create this market. It will take more than one buyer to get it done. Major buyers across the country will need to put their current benefit administration business up for bid using the type of market structure specifications that I outlined above. Buyers will need to move from hiring simple benefit administration services to hiring infrastructure vendors, entities that use today's computer-supported tool kits to truly create choice and improve care. Vertically integrated systems like ours will need to perform at levels that will set public standards for what is possible in that expanded environment of process improvement and continuous reengineering of care delivery and care.

This will happen only if buyers actually issue real requests for proposal (RFPs), develop and extend real specifications, and award the business and then use that approach to purchase care. I suspect that it will take a year or more to set up the RFPs and finish the vendor selection process and at least another year to implement the first major pieces of this new market approach. But I could be wrong. Some vendors and some buyers might move much more quickly once the market design end point is clearly defined as the new model. In other industries, change can be fairly rapid. Health care has been the exception—but health care hasn't had a new strategic direction or business model to deal with before now, so health care may have the potential to do much more than we had expected.

Businesses will need to negotiate prices with their vendors. As I noted earlier, this approach might work best if buyers evolve their health plan into a 401(k) clone, defined contribution model with their employees. Again, that's a very doable step, but people could decide to take a little or a lot of time to do it. And the model could be run just fine without that particular financial step.

If we set this model up well, the people covered by it will be able to select whether they want to receive care in an actual care system or in a virtual care system. People can decide who to use as caregivers. Prices for coverage and care can vary, based on patient choices. For the people who choose the virtual care system, benefit packages can still vary, giving people different price points for premiums. The infrastructure vendors then must give all the people who are covered far richer and more complete levels of information about their caregivers. Tracking performance in key areas will be an IV function that consumers need for making decisions. The IVs will also be accountable for providing patients with information that will help individuals make a number of very specific decisions about care. The original John Wennberg patient education modules about prostate surgery pioneered back in the late 1980s and breast surgery should be a model for those choices.[10] Patients need to understand the potential implications of their choices. Better choices result.

In keeping with that philosophy, providers in the new marketplace should expand the current approach to informed consent, to provide more specific information about either the specific surgeon or the care setting where the surgery is being done. Surgeons should provide the patient with a couple of key pieces of information, including how many times the surgeon has done that particular surgery before and what the outcomes of the surgery have been. Also, information about the historic success rate of the actual surgical unit could also be very relevant at that point. The death rate from coronary artery bypass surgery varies from as low as 1 percent to as high as 13 percent, depending on which hospital does the surgery.[11] Sharing that information with the patient on a timely basis might be useful for all parties. A 1,300 percent difference in the death rate for that surgery exists right now, and it is invisible. Making it visible will cause some patients to make safer choices. It would also, I'm sure, inspire some level of process improvement for the most problematic caregivers. If one goal of the IVs is to make currently available measurable results available directly to the patients at the most relevant point in patient decision making relevant to care, that could be a very good outcome.

Along those same lines, patient infection rates also vary significantly from hospital to hospital.[12] Those variations may get reported annually in an unlinked communication process, but they are typically not available to patients planning surgery. A well-structured, IV-run presurgery process could get that information as well to the relevant patients.

Performance improvement could happen. Patients need data. Patients also need selective interventions from an objective party when their care is outside of acceptable protocols. Patients definitely need both encouragement and support for healthy behaviors.

Again, someone needs to be hired to make all of that happen. It will not happen on its own. Once it does start to happen, I expect it to spread.

If the major buyers set up specifications for this new marketplace and then give that new market enough business to make it real, the new model will spill over to the rest of American health care fairly easily and very quickly. Smaller employers and individual purchasers of coverage can piggyback on the model and use it to buy their own coverage. Governmental units who purchase coverage for their employees could also use the model.

Various entitlement programs like Medicare and Medicaid could insist that their vendors make those same market functionalities available to their patients. Both Medicare and Medicaid have patients who very much need care management support. A workable and well-supported process of virtual case management should benefit both sets of patients.

And the uninsured need to be brought into this database and market model as well. Chapter Eleven deals with a proposal for universal coverage for this country. Universal coverage needs to be the next major reform for American health care. It's difficult to hold the entire care system accountable for care if the care-related data for fifty million Americans will not be part of that data base.

More on that later.

For now, the recommendation is that the major buyers need to change how coverage and care are purchased in the United States. The major buyers are the only folks who can do that quickly and well. It's time to make that happen.

8

Whom Should We Hire to Reform Our Health Care Infrastructure?

The only way we will build a new market-based care purchasing infrastructure in America will be if someone is hired to build it. I keep saying that because I believe it to be both an important point and very true.

The primary question we need to answer at this point is who exactly can and should be hired to do that job? What organization or business entities have the skill set, resources, in-place infrastructure, and market positioning to do that job? Who can and should be infrastructure vendors (IVs) hired to create those markets? The new market infrastructure we need will not spring into existence of its own volition, and it will not be created without a business model that makes fixing the existing infrastructure a viable business proposition with its own customers and its own revenue stream. Someone needs to do the heavy lifting to make those market settings real.

So who should that someone be? That's an extremely important question. Future success for American health care reform is highly dependent on getting that answer right.

Let me offer a possible list of infrastructure vendor candidates, or IVs.

Possible Infrastructure Vendors

1. *Government*. One possible IV candidate is the government—either state, federal or local government, depending on the specific IV strategy we select. That choice would require the government to collect and distribute data and to create a whole range of functionality relative to connectivity for customers and connectivity with caregivers.

2. *Major Provider Systems or Associations*. A second option to be the entity that realizes and refocuses the current nonsystematic health care infrastructure could be either major provider systems or local provider associations or confederations. The local hospital association or medical association in a given state might, for example, step up and take on those roles. So might a Mayo Clinic or a Cleveland Clinic or a large hospital system—for their respective service areas.

3. *Major Buyers*. A third option might be to have the major buyers themselves get together and form "purchasing coalitions" that also implement, manage, and maintain the whole array of infrastructure change processes and programs. Those coalitions could work together in various local markets to set up needed patient education and intervention, volume purchasing functions, data evaluation and communication functions, and interprovider connectivity functions. The buyers in each community could hire their own staff or some array of subcontractors to run those local health care markets.

4. *New Entities*. Another option might be to have brand new infrastructure management entities emerge—entrepreneurial organizations that put together a data flow and functionality that could reach out to the various buyer markets. One advantage of a well-funded, entirely new infrastructure reform entity is that it could reach out broadly between a wide range of local markets.

Buyer and caregiver coalitions are inherently pretty local. Most governmental units are pretty local as well. Even if government units were set up on a statewide level, one per state, having the state run the new markets could end up with the large buyers dealing with fifty separate state infrastructure vendors. That has its own set of issues.

By contrast, a brand new entity set up just to provide or arrange for these infrastructure reform services across all markets might be able to provide identical services in multiple states. That would be particularly true if the employers who hire that IV are all self-insured. Once insurance coverage or prepayment arrangements of any kind are introduced into the economic picture, and once smaller "insured" employers are brought into the overall new market purchasing process, the scalability and licensing status of those new vendors as "insurers" might be a bit more challenged.

5. *Existing Plans, Insurers, and Benefits Administrators*. In many ways, the most logical candidates to fill that infrastructure vendor role would be the organizations that are already providing many of those same services to many of the most likely customers. Those organizations include health plans, health insurance companies, and health benefit administrators. Those existing organizations already have in place much of the infrastructure needed to create both data flow and care improvement initiatives; the full set of patients' names, addresses, benefit choices, claims history, and relevant coverage and plan numbers are already in their databases.

Some of those existing benefit administration entities will find this proposal fascinating. Others will hate it, because it adds several challenging new dimensions to buyer expectations for both vendor functionality and performance. In particular, benefits administrators who have worked very hard over many years to eliminate any direct insurance risk or involvement in care improvement from their own business model may find the prospect of being accountable for care costs again to be a horrific idea. But others may love the idea and work hard to make it a reality.

Let me touch briefly on each of those options and then suggest some expectations that buyers and individual consumers should have for whoever is chosen to do that IV work.

1. Governmental Units as Potential Infrastructure Vendors

One obvious possible candidate for infrastructure reform vendors are governmental units. Local governments could certainly serve as the data-sharing vehicle for health care reform or as the infrastructure for population health improvement. It's possible to design a government-coordinated or government-led market reform model on paper.

Frankly, it's a lot harder to imagine either the state, federal, or local government actually taking on that full set of specific functional tasks in any consistent way in every city, town, and county—for example, persuading and helping local providers in local markets to form real or virtual teams to improve patient health and care outcomes in measurable ways. That is very heavy lifting, especially for an entity that has to be responsive to the political climate. This set of tasks, initiatives, operational infrastructures, and projects can be done well only if the total effort is well funded and well managed. Nongovernmental business entities are more likely to put in this kind of needed extra effort and investment in these new market areas because they expect to benefit economically over time for excellent performance. Governmental units are always cost centers, not profit centers. Cost centers naturally make very different decisions about investments. In most states, the infrastructure most likely to be used for those programs would be the programs that administer state Medicaid plans.

Existing state and local governmental units for the most part would not now have any in-place infrastructure or capabilities that would allow them to easily assume that role. That infrastructure would all have to be built. Government units would have to raise money to set up these programs. There's not a lot of unused government money sitting around in any governmental setting waiting to be invested in designing and building new health care administration infrastructure.

The federal government does have access to some of the necessary infrastructure through the Medicare and Medicaid databases.

However, the federal government, as well as state and local governments, could very easily run up against the issues we discussed earlier of having competing and contentious special interests and extremely powerful lobbying efforts pushing against what will sometimes be a lack of strong vision-empowered local or departmental governmental leadership—all compounded a bit by a lack of uniform and relevant expertise across many key administrative positions and operational functions.

A governmental approach would probably also have some difficulty being nimble—unable to change rapidly to meet the evolving need of buyers or patients as those needs are learned. The government in Britain, for example, which has had years of experience running a national health care system, has had difficulty trying to make some changes in their approach to the health care marketplace. Some very basic changes are taking more years to implement than the original NHS plans had targeted.[1]

Changing a bureaucracy is never easy. A governmental approach that requires formal processes to create actual operational rules might not respond quickly to new technology, new treatments, or new care approaches. Rule making in the government is not a nimble process; nor should it be. So although the government has some obvious theoretical attractions as a central organizing unit based on its potential objectivity, in many practical terms there are some real and probably insurmountable challenges to using the government as the primary infrastructure vendor if we want to achieve all of the care improvement goals I've outlined in this book.

2. Major Provider Systems or Associations as Potential Infrastructure Vendors

Major care providers, especially vertically integrated care systems like the Mayo Clinic, Cleveland Clinic, and Geisinger Medical Systems, could fill the role of infrastructure vendor in their communities. Building off a large, in-place, integrated provider database can be a very efficient way to get that total care integration and care improvement job done. There are not very many of these vertically integrated entities available in this country to do that job. Some of these entities, like Cleveland and Geisinger, have the tools necessary to provide financing; others, like the Mayo Clinic, do not, so they might well have to partner with an existing payer to offer a complete package to major buyers.

There are even fewer Kaiser Permanente–like organizations available with both care delivery and care financing functionality. Those few organizations have all of the tools necessary to both finance and provide care, but in limited geographic settings. Organizations like Kaiser Permanente will be important in the new health care marketplace as models of vertically integrated care, but will probably not be able, at least in the short run, to fill the rather large need for infrastructure vendors in many markets.

It will be even more difficult for local provider associations like hospital associations or medical associations that have neither the integrated provider database nor a care financing system to act as infrastructure vendors. Such groups would face the same issues as the other, better integrated vertical care systems, along with the financial burden of creating integrated databases and financing structures. These challenges would be compounded by the fact that the local internal politics of each provider association could often make objectivity in setting up meaningful comparative performance reporting a bit problematic. When legislatures now try to set up more complete provider reporting requirements, the entities lobbying most fiercely and most effectively against that reporting in most states do tend to be the various local providers and professional and trade associations.[2]

3. Buyer Coalitions as Potential Infrastructure Vendors

Buyers could choose to do the job themselves.

Major employers could decide to organize in local coalitions to fill in very directly as the data facilitators and program administrators.

Employers as a group could set up and run their own in-house or directly contracted care improvement and market facilitation processes.

So how well would the buyers do? In other areas, the operational trend is for companies to first become experts in setting up detailed purchasing specifications for the products and then to outsource the actual production of the good or service. In *The World Is Flat*, Thomas L. Friedman does of good job of explaining how that outsourcing works, both locally and internationally.[3] The notion of major buyers taking the exact opposite direction for health care and going from developing detailed specifications to directly delivering detailed services is not likely to fit into the strategic agenda of most major companies. But it can be done.

The particular skill sets and administrative systems needed to set up a health care market infrastructure aren't all in place now in very many, if any, American corporate human resource departments. But hiring could be done, and local buyer coalitions could put in place a whole new buyer-owned infrastructure for care management, employee education, data collection, data reporting, and quality improvement.

The overall prospect of having buyer-led and buyer-administered approaches to best care and care system organization that vary across each market by employer after employer might be a problem for some people relative to overall health care reform agendas. Having separate coalitions in a great many markets could be a challenge, particularly for multistate employers, and the work of somehow organizing and setting up a single national buyer coalition could be unbelievably and unacceptably time-consuming and problematic.

There are scale issues as well. How big would that buyer-run infrastructure need to be? Where would it be located? Who exactly would own it? Working together as a group to jointly purchase services gives employers great economic leverage. Working as a group to actually deliver those same explicit services is a whole different picture.

One piece of relevant history in that regard might be derived from a sizable buyer coalition that formed a decade or so ago in

Minnesota.[4] In the early days, when the buyers worked together to function as a "purchasing pool with clear specifications," the coalition did really well. The entire operation was outsourced. The specifications for the overall project came jointly from the employers, which gave them a lot of leverage, because they all agreed on one set of specifications. The coalition then negotiated a great deal as a buyer to rent a local health plan infrastructure to implement those specifications. Several local infrastructures bid on the business. One was selected, and great progress was made. That model received national recognition.[5]

In that original model, the entire administrative and provider network infrastructure was farmed out by the buyers. The buyers purchased care reform instead of managing or administering any part of care. The original buying coalition staff was tiny, made up mainly of specification administrators. It worked.

When that same coalition later changed strategies and decided to "self-administer" the program, the challenges of functionality were totally different. In the new self-administered model, the buyers had to spend their time on a whole different set of mundane issues. Administrative functions became a high priority. Trying to get credible levels of performance data became a problem. In my opinion, economic leverage diminished significantly, and the group went from being the largest and best leveraged buying coalition in America to simply being the "fifth largest health plan" in Minnesota. Doing it yourself can be a hard way to go.

That particular buyer decision to insource reform rather than outsource had impacts that others might want to study. It's not easy for buyers as a coalition to become the actual frontline health care administrators or process improvement managers. It's very workable to set the specifications and then hire someone with great competence to get the job done.

Unit costs of care can also be a longer-term issue when that insourcing decision is made. Even very large employers or coalitions generally don't have enough volume to purchase care at optimal levels from each of the caregivers in all of the various markets needed for the infrastructure to perform as a real low-cost network. A large employer deciding to "self-contract" for care would need contracts with thousands of caregivers. Maybe tens of thousands, depending on the geographic marketplace that the employer operates in. It can be a lot easier for employers to hire someone with higher volume levels to do all of that contracting work rather than to do the work directly.

4. Brand New Entities as Potential Infrastructure Vendors

Another option that I suspect will surface if buyers decide to set up an open request for proposal (RFP) process to hire IVs is new entities that form in response to that RFP opportunity. I would also expect to see a number of existing entities change their business model in response to the RFPs. Capitalistic innovators of multiple ilks could well respond in quantity if the buyers open the RFP process to all interested bidders. Health care is the fastest growing industry in America.[6] We could expect to see a lot of organizations look hard at the opportunity to become an IV.

The total response to the new RFPs might be really interesting. Organizations who now provide care management services, like free-standing disease management companies, might, for example, choose to build on their existing data platforms to add on the expanded functionality needed for consumer-patients to make benefit package choices and to actually pay providers and process claims. The care management firms already run profiles of patients based on computerized claims databases.[7] At this point, those firms generally have little involvement with the patients' actual care providers—they work more to influence patient behavior.[8] But those organizations would probably love having more leverage to influence the actual providers of care.

The challenges would be, obviously, for the care management firms to set up a provider payment process with sufficient functionality to price and pay claims as well as maintain customer service records, member eligibility records, and actuarial data. They also would have the challenge of building the software systems required by this market model. The market model I have described here, based on interactive databases available through richly functional web sites, depends heavily on information technology (IT).

Because of the emphasis on IT, I would expect to see software businesses that already do extensive health care work looking at the opportunity to build on existing functionality to expand their capability to serve as IVs. These vendors might choose to enter into the second round of bidding, particularly once the first round of bids and implementations defines the new market. Banks and other financial transaction entities might feel similar temptations. There's a lot of money flowing through health care. Organizations that handle money for a living will be interested.

Other vendors that might be interested in bidding on IV RFPs are organizations founded from scratch simply to do that work—with both for-profit and not-for-profit community-based models possible.

As I said, the response to the RFP process could be fascinating. We could see IV bids of many forms and shapes.

5. Existing Health Plans, Insurers, and Administrators as Potential Infrastructure Vendors

The other potential vendors who generally seem to already have the most complete array of in-place capability for facilitating data access, assembling care networks, tracking and reporting care performance, and then taking financial accountability for the direct economic consequences of care are the various entities that function today as health plans, health insurance companies, or health benefit administrators.

Most of the infrastructure needed to administer the coverage portion of the new market is already in place—well tested and well staffed. The challenge, as I noted earlier, would be to get many of those entities to expand that financial and care management functionality to serve as a next-generation health plan, an infrastructure vendor that functions as an agent of the buyers and the patients to directly influence and reform specific key elements of the existing infrastructure of care.

Health plans are fairly likely to already have many of the computer systems, customer volumes, provider networks, administrative staffing, and internal resources to do much of that job. Up to now, however, existing health plans and benefits administrators have not all been willing to take on those market reform roles. Some cost containment and care management functions currently exist, but they haven't been the primary product of the plans or the administrators. For the new market of informed choices to exist, the role for the plans or plan equivalents would need to change in ways that can meet the new infrastructure vendor care performance specifications set by major buyers.

That new plan role can build on the extremely convenient fact that significant levels of data about patients and their care already flow through every plan's computers, as does the actual cash used to pay the providers. Money talks. That's why the data is already there. Today's benefit administration cash flow already creates that data flow. As we discussed back in Chapters Two and Three, it is the claims payment process that is already fully in place today that creates the current nonvoluntary, economically mandatory constant flow of essential care-related data from providers to payers.

Mandatory is the key concept here. I can tell you from years of trying in various settings, it's often really hard to get sufficient data on any topic or area of performance from voluntary data sources. Even the best-intentioned voluntary data compilation efforts generally fall short. If cash isn't involved, the priority level for providers to send in data may not be high. Any entity completely external to the current cash flow of health care that tries to start from scratch to collect equivalent and timely care-related data through some new voluntary (or even legally involuntary) reporting mechanism is obviously going to face a logistical and economic challenge. The task of trying to create and work with a primarily voluntary flow of data is likely to be extremely challenging.

Setting up a whole new health care data flow outside of the actual provider payment process might be possible at a future point in time when all providers have installed operational, uniform electronic medical records (EMRs). Connecting a world of functioning EMRs would be relatively easy. But building a pure provider-based data set will be virtually impossible until that happens.

For now, in the short term, the claims payment process wins as the easiest to use and most likely to succeed data flow. Directly siphoning the relevant care data off the existing health care payment cash flow mechanism is, for a number of obvious reasons, the most dependable short-term approach to long-term data availability, data consistency, and data accessibility.

In the ideal world outlined in Chapter Six, the "plan equivalent," or infrastructure vendor, would need to go beyond the traditional payer role with its traditional data storage strategies to build the kinds of computer systems that would continuously access and scan the community aggregate personal health record database and then format that data in accessible ways to help each patient and caregiver served by the plan get easy electronic access to needed information. The IV needs to facilitate data access so each patient can make informed choices about his caregivers and his care and so that each caregiver can have a better sense of the total care needs of each patient.

The infrastructure vendors could and should compete with each other based on the measurable results they achieve in improving the quality and cost of care, and based on the quality and usefulness of the infrastructure they each provide to help individual patients make informed choices about their care.

How Would the Infrastructure Vendors Function?

Each new infrastructure vendor will need to track care by key diagnosis and then work with the care providers to ensure that, for at least the five major chronic conditions, optimal care is being delivered.

Infrastructure vendors will be able to achieve those goals for buyers in various ways. Some organizations, like ours at Kaiser Permanente, are so tightly integrated now—from physicians to pharmacists to hospitals—that the care improvement agenda can be inherent to the structure. Other plan equivalents could offer tightly contracted networks of care, with contractual relationships relative to care improvement. Some may offer newly exclusive or inclusive networks of providers who agree to work under contract to comply with care protocols and performance expectations.

Other infrastructure vendors will work more through the patients, advising the caregivers and simultaneously counseling the patients, connecting with both providers and patients through the telephone and computer, and using those tools to significantly influence the delivery of care.

As I noted earlier, the existence of some variety in approaches will be a good thing. Different approaches will create a much richer learning environment, and time will tell which approach or design best meets the needs of each market and each community.

A key for care performance will be measurement—real measurement—of second heart attacks, crisis-level congestive heart failure attacks, and emergency asthma attacks. The buyers need to require their IVs to set clear standards and goals for care improvement in each of those major performance areas and then use the new community-standard personal health record (PHR) database and a network of computerized disease registries to track, measure, and reward care outcomes.

Those IVs that are plan equivalents will need to tap into that community PHR database, assemble networks, track and report performance data, set up a patient-focused Internet infrastructure, facilitate e-counseling sessions for patients and caregivers, and set up internal reward systems for caregivers and teams of caregivers.

Three Payment Options

How should the IVs and care networks be paid? There are three payment options: prepayment, a mix of prepayment and self-insurance, and pure self-insurance.

1. Prepayment

Prepayment means that the buyer negotiates a flat price with the IV for the full costs of covered care, with a number of care improvement performance expectations written into the contract. If the performance specifications are clear and initial data is completely available, and if all provider and infrastructure performance is entirely transparent, then a pure prepayment model offers the simplest and cleanest payment approach. How would that work? It's a pretty basic model. A pure prepayment model IV would negotiate a fixed price to provide each level of coverage and care to a defined population of covered persons. In that model, a fixed annual cost per covered person would be paid by the buyer, and the IV would be responsible for giving employees choices of benefit packages and providers and for achieving the specific care performance goals and infrastructure performance goals, while living within that negotiated prepayment amount.

The market result of that pure prepayment approach is not dissimilar to Wal-Mart or Target buying entire TVs from a TV vendor for a fixed price. Wal-Mart does not buy one electronic part of a TV from one electronics vendor in Korea and another physical part of the TV from a separate vendor in Thailand and then have either Wal-Mart staff or the customers put all the parts together in Tennessee to create a TV. Wal-Mart buys TVs, not parts. Wal-Mart sets the specifications for the entire TV and then buys the final product intact and assembled from each TV vendor. The TV prices are negotiated as a package. The price is preset. Wal-Mart doesn't buy cost-plus TVs. Wal-Mart doesn't allow any TV vendor to say, "We'll buy our chips in one place and our cords in another and our screens in another, and then we'll add up the costs and charge Wal-Mart whatever those vendors charge us, with a little markup for our overhead and TV assembly functions. We hope the price of the parts will be low—and we'll negotiate to keep them low, but if we fail to keep those costs down, hey, it's not our fault. We will just document all of those costs fully and we'll charge Wal-Mart whatever the new cost is."

I don't know about you, but I don't think I could personally sell that deal to Best Buy, Target, JCPenney, or Wal-Mart. That's not how big companies buy TVs. But it is how American companies buy health care.

In health care, if an IV has a specification obligation calling for a specific targeted reduction in heart attacks and asthma crisis, and sells the employer an entire health care package guaranteeing that outcome for a fixed monthly price—with full transparency on care performance and outcomes—then the health care vendor, like the TV vendor, would need to use its own internal expertise to bring the entire product to market for the negotiated fixed price. That approach pays the provider network set up by the IV for the total results of care—not just the total cost of all units of care. In a prepaid model, it's up to the IV to manage the internal cost structure to meet the negotiated price. I'll discuss ways IVs can do that in a few pages. Competency for IVs in the area of cost management will be extremely important.

2. Prepaid and Self-Insurance Mix

Other payment options exist. A second way for employers to buy health care in the context of that new IV-administered market model might be to buy care for certain patients (like people with diabetes or asthma) on a prepaid, fixed-cost basis, while buying care for other categories of patients on a self-insured, unit-by-unit basis. Cancer care, for example, might be an expense that is passed directly from the IV to the buyers on a self-insured, fee-for-service payment approach. The buyers would simply pay for whatever the costs of cancer care turned out to be.

Why use self-insurance in the payment mix? A lot of employers prefer to self-insure their health care expenses rather than buy insured coverage. Self-insurance means that the employer takes the risk of care expenses and simply hires an administrator to pay the claims using the employer's money. When no one is really managing care, self-insurance can make a lot of sense. Why pay someone else for a risk assumption function you can do yourself for less money? That equation changes a bit if care management becomes a purchased service and ends up being done well. An IV that manages costs against prenegotiated payment levels is different from an insurer who takes risks and charges an "experience-based" premium. One role is active. The other is passive. Self-insurance can easily replace the passive role.

It's possible to mix and match self-insurance with an insured product.

For example, it doesn't make much sense to self-insure a fee-for-service chronic care. What we know about patients with chronic diseases is that they need continuous, ongoing care to prevent their disease from developing and progressing, and we know what that care should look like. It makes sense to prepay for that care, based on buyer specifications. Prepayment might involve negotiating a flat monthly fee with the IV for each diabetic patient—with a higher payment for patients with comorbidities.

At the same time, all direct costs for some levels of acute care could be passed directly on to the buyer at a self-insured, fee-for-service payment level. The payment for acute care could be fee-based, and the payment for chronic care could be patient-based. Diabetic care, by contrast, might then be prepaid, with the buyer paying a prenegotiated fixed total monthly cost per patient with diabetes. The plan IV's job in that case would be to work in the context of the prepayment cash flow to set up whatever care networks and care protocols are needed to achieve the care improvement goals negotiated with the employer.

It could be a very good strategy to pay for chronic care results using a slightly different approach from the acute care services. That prepayment calculation for chronic care patients can be more than a little complicated when patients have multiple comorbidities that include both acute and chronic conditions. But it can be done.

Again, relative to the acute care issues, if the individual patients are each making informed choices about their oncologists, orthopedic surgeons, or urinary tract caregivers based on very visible cost difference and performance data, that data flow and purchasing process will all by itself both improve the quality of care and reduce the cost. Creating and managing that data flow about acute care procedures and services needs to be part of the specifications that the new IV plan equivalent must meet in order to be hired by the employer, even for the care levels that might continue to be self-insured by the employer.

3. Pure Self-Insurance

A third payment approach that could be used by larger buyers in the context of this market model is just to continue using pure self-insurance for at least part of their covered population, with the buyer taking the full financial risk for the cost of care for those particular people. If that model is used, it would probably work best as an overlay on an existing IV structure that already uses prepayment approaches with most of its customers and providers, so the basic incentives of prepayment and the experience of living within a premium limit for other customers establishes and sculpts the IV's and the providers' basic approach to care even for the self-insured patients.

In this self-insured, service-only payment approach, it will be important for the buyer to also pay the IV for the various additional functions needed to manage population care and provider performance management. It could also be important for the self-insured buyers to participate proportionately in any financial reward system set up by the IV to encourage caregivers to achieve optimal goals in areas like prevention, health improvement, and complication reduction. The contract between the buyer and the plan equivalent could spell out both expected performance standards and the costs of care management programs and incentives.

The key is to hire someone to do that work, whether they be prepaid or fee paid.

As noted earlier, someone needs to be accountable for population health improvement, or that improvement will not occur. Someone has to be financially rewarded or penalized for population health improvement successes and failures, or those efforts will not be funded or operationalized. It takes cash flow to create economic incentives, and any economic incentive model works only if someone is directly impacted financially by the cash flow. Leading, coordinating, organizing, and operating that process is a task that needs to be assigned to someone whose resource flow is directly affected by their performance in those areas.

We've already proved that real reform does not happen without that overarching organizing factor. Health plans performed some of those functions for a number of years, but that initial effort to actually "manage care" softened quite a bit over the past half decade for most plans. The trend for most buyers has been to go back to pure fee-for-service care with negotiated discounts and little or no influence on care delivery in most areas of care.[9] Nonmanaged fee-for-service, self-insured medicine was the product that buyers decided to purchase from the late 1990s through 2006,[10] so that was the product that existed. And that was the product that facilitated and enabled the absence of any meaningful process reengineering or quality reform in American health care.

Hiring an IV to deliver care using a prepaid fixed price puts the full cost pressure very directly on the IV. Using a shared risk approach dilutes that focus a bit. But the model can still work. It's time for buyers to demand, specify, and then purchase a different product from pure insurance administration functions. The new model needs to improve care in measurable ways. Buyers should insist that their IVs give larger clients in-depth data on their own employee population's costs and performance in key areas, with a focus on changing the cost burden systematically for the higher-cost health conditions. Buyers should also partner with their vendors to change employee behaviors, educate patients about best care, and influence local care providers to use best practices and optimal efficiency.

This is not a new idea for most industries. In the manufacturing world, big companies often partner with their suppliers in highly cooperative ways to improve the overall production process. The Japanese pioneered a process called *keiretsu*[11] that actually created partnerships between Japanese manufacturers and their key vendors relative to production processes and prices. Similar levels of close cooperation make sense in purchasing a health package—as enlightened and networked buyers work closely with health vendors to persuade patients to use the best care providers and to practice good health habits.

Communitywide Data Is Needed

Buyers also need to strongly support the overall effort to create a communitywide, aggregated, personal health record (PHR) database. Patient privacy needs to be a top priority of that agenda. The PHR database should simultaneously create total privacy for individual patients and total transparency for individual providers. Patients need to know that their own personal health records are available only to them and to the caregivers or advisors they authorize to receive and use that data. Individual privacy is an absolute priority. But individual privacy should not block or prevent a separate and patient-anonymous set of communitywide provider performance transparency. We need community data so each community can know how well it is doing on asthma care or congestive heart failure in ways that allow and encourage the systematic improvement of that care.

Health vendors also need access to that data on an aggregate level by provider, so that performance tracking becomes possible in a highly credible and convenient way.

Buyers should also insist that their IVs facilitate both "virtual consults" by individual patients and the use of evidence-based care in systematic ways. Every health vendor should be a participant in community health improvement initiatives, with buyers insisting on those initiatives as a condition of purchasing care, coverage, and administrative services from the vendor.

The potential savings are huge. We could cut crisis-level asthma attacks by 80 percent.[12] We could cut heart attacks to a level a third lower than the general population.[13] We could cut the number of people whose kidneys fail by a third.[14] Those wins are all possible, but only if we use the tools of a common provider number, an electronic data flow, comparative provider performance, an Internet-enabled information share, clearly communicated medical protocols, best practice, improved patient wellness-related behaviors, and the right cash incentives to improve both care and care outcomes.

So now is the time to take on that agenda. As I have said repeatedly, this particular revolution needs to be buyer-led. Buyers have great skill levels for purchasing almost every other significant area of expense—so it's time to extend that expertise to the purchase of coverage and care.

9

Next Steps and Expectations

We should not expect that every element of this new market model can be put in place on Day One. It will take several years to get all these pieces in place. But a lot can be done in Year One and Year Two—particularly if we have a really clear sense of where we want this process to end up. We need to know on Day One exactly what we expect the fully functional future versions of this new model to be, and then we need to understand exactly how far we can go in Year One, Year Two, Year Three, and the years after that.

We should expect that the rollout of the new model will be in pieces, not done all in one fell swoop as a fully formed operation. That's just common sense. This new market model can and should be set up in incremental stages. It doesn't need to deal with every single medical condition on Day One. We really don't even need to deal with every condition in the first year. In fact, it probably makes the most sense to set the entire process up to focus initially on just the five key chronic diseases and then evolve over a defined period of time, as data availability and system functionality allows, to include other medical conditions. Remember the data. The major opportunities are in the chronic diseases. Let's start there.

Some patience on the part of buyers will be required while the initial retail marketplace quality and price data set is established. But if the vendors clearly spell out their multiyear plans to the buyers, it's possible to get the whole process underway very soon with a specific multiyear end point both clearly in mind and well defined for each type and category of care.

The starting point for all players would be to have solid baseline data on current levels of success in key areas of care for at least their chronic care patients as quickly as possible. For the major employers who would be the initial purchasers of those services, the baseline data could and should be specific to their own employee population. For smaller employers, the baseline data on those conditions could be community-level data and risk pool specific data for each infrastructure vendor.

Specific Quantifiable Goals

Once baseline data are established, the next step in the process is to set specific, quantifiable goals for care improvement—fewer heart attacks, fewer asthma crises, and so forth. In the request for proposal (RFP) process, each market infrastructure vendor should make its sales pitch to the buyer based on the specific goals that each vendor intends to achieve in each of those areas. The economic benefit to the employer of achieving each goal can and should be outlined by each vendor in bidding on the business. In a competitive market setting, the infrastructure vendor (IV) bidding process will also evolve, with vendor creativity about how to achieve each of those measurable goals an essential part of the new market model product development process.

An extremely important evaluation step for each buyer will be to carefully review the virtual connectivity tool kit that the chosen market infrastructure vendor will use to achieve each of those communication and care management goals. Initially, those tool kits will vary a lot from vendor to vendor. As noted above, that's actually a good thing, because experimentation in improving population health will help make everyone smarter. No one has all the answers today. But those answers are all knowable. And very smart people will come up with very creative approaches when those approaches lead to sales and revenue for both the market infrastructure vendors and the providers of care.

Keep in mind that there will be more than one possible path to each of the desired outcomes. I've emphasized using computerized data and various levels of electronic connectivity to create "virtual vertical integration." However, a vendor in a particular market might rely heavily on directly contacting and educating patients. That could be a very successful approach for buyers whose primary users of health care are categories of patients who may not be comfortable with using the Internet for their daily business. Another vendor might offer creative benefit designs combined with a really effective patient information web site.

No matter which IV is chosen, the better approaches will be either virtually or vertically integrated, computer supported, and will use a multidisciplinary team of providers working in full partnership with each other and the patients to achieve those goals.

The key here is not that a single best approach exists, but that the vendor selected by the employer very directly takes on the job of changing health outcomes and improving health in a reasonable and effective way for each of the buyer's clearly defined and specified care category performance areas. Measurement of performance can be done using both internal IV data and the new standardized personal health record (PHR) database to compare current numbers with both past data and communitywide data. With the emergence of the new PHR databases as a tracking mechanism and the support of highly motivated buyers, a number of alternative vendors will create innovative ways of getting good measurements developed and then getting the needed care improvement job done.

Standards for Population Health

Buyers need to set standards and goals relative to population health for their chronic care patients. Figure 7.1 in Chapter Seven includes hypothetical examples of these. Buyers need to say, "We need an asthma crisis reduction of 30 percent over two years. Your payment as a vendor is dependent on our patients reaching that goal." Negotiations on those specific payments and prices need to take place between vendors and buyers, with very clear goals in mind.

Also, as part of the specification-setting process, the buyer needs to say, "We need our employees to have real data about provider performance. We want a dozen to two dozen patient-relevant data points on your web site about breast cancer detection rates, breast cancer surgery five-year survival rates, and so on. We want that information available electronically to our patients by next July. Part of your job as our IV—our care delivery master contractor—is to provide us and our employees with that data."

In the past, that level of data would not have been available for any of those purposes. Please don't underestimate how big a change could happen in health care if the IVs do their jobs well. Before the PHR database was a gleam in anyone's eye, real data about comparative cancer survival rates were, at best, available on very rare occasions from tiny local research projects run in isolated settings and focused on a finite number of patients for a very finite period of time. In the new data world, that type of data should be available to patients through a continuously improving set of measurements and reviews.

At this point in the RFP process, the upcoming initial challenge for the health improvement master contractor will be to explain clearly to the buyer how and when specific needed data will be gathered and how it will then be used to give consumers needed information about their care choices, and providers needed information about care status.

This is a whole new way of looking at the purchase of care: buying results and not just processes. The five chronic conditions that run up most of our health care costs are obviously very logical and high-potential initial targets for this new approach to purchasing.

The basic concept of this approach is that it's time to buy and sell care for our most expensive categories of care and patients in a business model where providers work together to create both best care and real efficiency and effectiveness in care delivery. Asthma care, diabetes care, heart and congestive heart failure (CHF) care should all be available through a market model that guarantees appropriate levels of consumer choice and provider teamwork.

Each vendor can figure out how to pay and incent the caregivers in their network to provide the most effective management of that care. There should be transparency for the buyers about that process, but the buyer would probably be better off not micromanaging those approaches. When Apple buys a chip from a vendor, Apple sets up explicit specs on the chip but generally doesn't micromanage how the chip vendor deals with its own employees or its own subcontractors. That's a good model to follow.

Data-Supported, Informed Choices

How we purchase care can have a major impact on the chronic care patients who incur over 70 percent of our total health care costs. That's a fairly obvious opportunity. What has been less obvious is that a better designed health care marketplace can improve outcomes and costs for nonchronic diseases as well. Patients with various acute care problems and diseases also very much need a far better market model at the retail level.

How can that be done? With data, clear expectations, and benefits packages that incent the use of cost-effective care providers. We need to evolve over the next couple of years into a new, electronically supported health care marketplace for patients with acute care needs, where individual consumers can make informed health care choices between health care providers. Patients who need knee surgery should be able to know the relative success rates of various orthopedic surgeons. Patients with lung cancer should know the relative survival rates and the care strategies for each oncologist or oncology group available. We will all be better off as patients and caregivers if those kinds of performance statistics are known to everyone. Caregivers will also be more able to improve their own performance based on solid and relevant information about the relative comparative success levels of their fellow practitioners. Everybody is going to benefit from a marketplace of informed caregiver and care option choices. The value is particularly relevant when performance data is linked to the cost of key units of care. That approach is described in more detail below.

Having the data-rich marketplace needed to support individual consumers' choice is highly dependent on actually having aggregate access to the data embedded in the claims-based computer files. If there is an aggregated PHR database assembled by each community and if that database is made available to all payers, providers, patients, vendors, and buyers in ways that completely and totally protect individual patient confidentiality, then that database can be the foundation for key items of performance data needed to measure and report caregiver and community performance in quite a few areas. Very large carriers or health plans will have their own statistically credible database in many markets, and some can use their own internal database to do this work. But if we also want smaller players to be able to compete as IVs for the health business of the buyers, a "public" version of that community PHR database will need to be available to all possible vendors and users. That database will create the needed foundation for possible new levels of care improvement competition.

We could and should also create web sites with both hard data and direct communications from the caregivers. There should be bloglike feedback mechanisms for patients in the new market model. One IV value improvement feature might be for each IV to host a "certified patient experience blog" that ensures that only patients who had actually been treated by a physician would be allowed to comment in that doctor's blog about that doctor's performance. Otherwise, without that level of screening by some credible service, a percentage of Internet comments about physicians that are most interesting or most persuasive may actually have no real experiential validity. Sometimes people lie on open blogs. Very creative people pretend to be telling real-life stories on some blogs. That can be very interesting reading, but it's not the best source of credible data about actual care or real-life experiences. I've seen situations where it appears that competitors lie openly about other caregivers to move patients. The logical result of those lies isn't better care. A "certified" patient experience blog that is well administered by an IV could be a real value for patients. That's one possible IV role among many. The IV needs to be a skilled web host for multiple categories of relevant information. Providers also need their own web space. A team of knee surgeons might note on their web site: "The community success rate on knee surgery is 47 percent. We have a 65 percent success rate. That's because we each evaluate each other's surgery every week. Team care is good care. Use us." Or words to that effect. You get the idea. Caregivers should be encouraged by the IV to give patients information that can help them make better-informed choices. One of the beauties of the Internet is that any provider self-claims that are inaccurate stand a very high likelihood of being contradicted on the Internet by direct patient input. The Internet creates amazing levels of both transparency and information distribution. That reality will only grow as time goes on, so we should incorporate it directly into the design of our infrastructure reform in the most useful and enlightened ways.

We've already seen very interesting performance comparisons and comments on care categories like eye surgery.

We've also recently seen comparative quality data used in an attempt to lure American patients overseas. JCAHO-accredited hospitals in India, for example, now offer to do heart surgery for half the cost of some American care sites at measurably higher levels of quality than a number of American care sites.[1] It would be a shame if the only level of effective data-based quality competition in health care turned out to be international Internet trolling on the web for American patients by offshore hospitals.

Setting up a local competitive market for key areas of care will benefit everyone in America.

Cost Competition Is Needed

Quality is one issue. Cost is another. We need real competition in both areas. Ideally, providers and infrastructure vendors will both offer levels of cost competition. Infrastructure vendors will compete with each other based on premium levels for insured groups and based on claims payment cost levels for self-insured buyers. At the provider level, fees will need to be publicly known and easily available to consumers making cost-conscious choices. The infrastructure vendors will all have their own negotiated prices with each care provider, so the infrastructure vendor web sites will need to make that specific provider cost information available on the web in very easy-to-use ways as needed by the consumers who want to make price-conscious decisions about care.

Some people now argue for a communitywide aggregated web site for provider cost information that contains all the pricing information, including free market prices and IV negotiated prices, for all buyers and all providers. A total data load approach that lists all prices for all payers for all services is actually not operationally optimal for patients or consumers, for the simple reason that not all patients using the web site would be eligible for all prices. People with coverage through a specific IV or health plan will have access only to the specific prices negotiated by that IV or plan. As a result, the individual IV web sites will generally be the best and most useful source of patient-relevant price data for their own customer-patients.

For example, a given hospital might have negotiated six different prices with six different IVs or health plans for chest scans. In that situation, the only directly and personally relevant cost numbers for that consumer are the actual and specific prices negotiated by that consumer's IV with each provider. Those prices need to be easily available to the consumer when the consumer is a member of that plan. Knowing the prices available to members of other plans with a given care provider might be interesting, but since those other prices are only available to the members of that plan, having all prices from all IVs on one web site might be extremely confusing.

Individual consumers who want to shop for the best plan will find the new world of web data to be an incredibly useful tool.

If consumers with appropriately designed cost-sharing benefit packages know both the relative care outcomes and the exact relevant costs within their plan for each available caregiver, the marketplace for care can far more directly reward best care and maximize care value. Buyers who select plans should insist that capability be part of the infrastructure offered by the plan, using both internal plan data and the overall performance data available through the aggregated PHR database.

Benefit Design Will Be Extremely Important

The primary goal of benefit plan design for IVs should be to have the patients appropriately incented and supported to make the right decisions about coverage, care systems, caregivers, and care. Care is the magical point in the whole process. We absolutely do not want a patient with asthma to not fill a needed prescription because of how we designed the benefit package. That would be a mistake. We also do not want a marketplace that insulates doctors who charge $100 for a basic office visit from market pressures that could and should force the price down to $60 or $80. We do want a market that encourages caregivers to set up simple, efficient, and low-cost care sites in supermarkets and retail centers that might offer a $40 office visit—and we want to encourage each health care provider to use care staff more creatively and effectively to get a higher-quality outcome with more efficiency and lower cost.

Tiered benefits can also be useful. Tiered benefits are used very effectively now with prescription drugs, where low copayments are assigned to generic drugs to encourage patients to use the generic version.[2] Tiered benefits have been used a bit less successfully for hospital coverage.[3] Tiers have been less successful for hospitals because the linkage between cost and value hasn't been as logical and apparent. Some of the higher-cost hospitals are legitimately higher in cost because they provide needed specialty services and care unavailable elsewhere in the community. Charging the patients more when that unique level of specialty care is urgently needed doesn't fit the philosophy of using benefit design to incent both smart and wise choices, because the patients in that situation often have no other local low-cost choice for that level of specialty care. A better benefit design would be to charge the patient who uses the higher-cost hospital more only if the more expensive service received at the higher-cost hospital was also a service readily available at a local lower-cost hospital. That service specific approach requires a more careful benefit design, but it fits the goal of actually incenting appropriate choices quite a bit better. It isn't a simple issue, however.

If the consequence of tertiary hospitals in a given community losing their less complex and more lucrative patients is to force the price even higher for their less-subsidized secondary or tertiary care patients, the cost of care could go up for the entire local risk pool of patients. So tiering hospital benefits should be done only after a very clear analysis of the likely impact of patient movement on the total cost of community care.

Benefit design at that more sophisticated level requires a well-informed and highly skilled IV working in partnership with the buyer. The buyer partnership on those issues is key. If the employer says, "I would like my employees to use the less expensive drugs and the less expensive hospital when quality is the same, but I don't want any real financial incentives or penalties used to encourage my employees to make those low-cost choices," then the vendor is at a significant disadvantage relative to influencing patient choices. Partnerships on benefit design are needed to get optimal results.

If the marketplace is set up so that consumers can make informed, data-supported decisions about their caregivers—and if the consumers have benefit packages that do not stand as a barrier to needed care but definitely do require the consumer to pay more to choose a more expensive caregiver—and if all other factors remain equal—then providers in that marketplace would be much more sensitive to their comparative price point and the market would reward the better, lower-priced performers with additional business.

Link Payments to Performance

In summary, the new market model for health care should directly link payment with desired performance, so that caregivers who perform well are rewarded with business and money. As I keep saying, the current marketplace for care has almost nine thousand billing codes for units of care, and not one billing code for a cure. It also has zero billing codes for improved patient health or for any form of results or outcomes. To make matters worse, consumers purchase care in a marketplace where there is no comparative data about caregiver performance, success levels, or cost. The RAND study and the IOM studies have shown that our current marketplace for care is inconsistent, wasteful, undependable, and sometimes dangerous for patients. It's the most expensive model for health care in the world, and caregivers are not rewarded in any way for being efficient or cost-competitive. Patients receiving care in America far too often suffer from frequent care linkage deficiencies, and patients with multiple health conditions too often find themselves with multiple, uncoordinated caregivers.

It's not the system we want or should have.

We need buyers who do real volume purchasing and can set up relevant specifications, beginning with desired care outcomes for the five chronic diseases that trigger most health care costs in this country. We need buyers who recognize the reality that our patients with heart disease, diabetes, and asthma need consistent team care. We need buyers who are willing to buy that care as a package from people who assemble that care as a package and then deliver performance in actually improving that care.

Health care needs vendors who are prepaid for each person with diabetes for total coordinated diabetic care—vendors who set up and meet specific performance standards both for diabetic care processes and diabetic care outcomes.

Building and using infrastructure vendor specifications should become an art, a science, and a core competency for major buyers. Infrastructure management should be a business model and a profession. Appropriately incented care for chronic diseases should be an expectation, not an exception. Infrastructure vendors need to set those incentive programs up in ways that achieve measurable results.

How Many Infrastructure Vendors Do We Need?

That raises an important question. How many separate infrastructure reform vendors would a single buyer need to use? Not very many. Most markets will probably end up with only a few vendors who will be able to take on that full scope of services and have a full network of providers under contract. It's probably a good idea for major buyers not to become entirely reliant on a single infrastructure vendor for all of their employees. It's also a good idea not to have so many vendors that the data from each vendor becomes statistically irrelevant and the administrative overhead of managing the array of vendors becomes excessive. Having a couple of vendors in key markets—maybe experimenting with vendors who offer different care management tools and models—would allow for internal competition and would give the employer a sense of comparative performance. Having too many infrastructure reform vendors could become complex and make useful comparisons less valid.

In each case, giving the employees a choice of vertically integrated systems versus virtually integrated systems is a good foundational practice that can create a great competition relative to performance outcomes and cost. The ultimate organizational goal of health care is provider teamwork and mutual achievement. Any choice model that excludes local vertically integrated systems as a possible choice for employees is a step backward from the ultimate goals of American care system evolution.

This new market model will happen only if influential buyers decide to make it real. It can be done. All the necessary pieces exist. But they won't be assembled until the market emerges and starts to make purchases. And then it will take a couple of years to get all the key ingredients in place.

Once this approach is fairly well in place, by the way, it will be a huge blessing for the various government programs that desperately need costs controlled for those very same categories of patients. Medicare can't lead the way, but there's no reason Medicare can't be a very fast follower once the care improvement model has proven its value.

So it's time to put a new health care marketplace in place. We need vendors who sell both population health improvement and process reengineering for care delivery. We need a data-rich, choice-based health care marketplace facilitated by highly skilled infrastructure reform vendors. We need to pay those vendors for the success they achieve. We need to put each of those reforms in place sequentially, starting with hiring the IVs and following with a fast focus on those extremely expensive chronic care cost levels. We need to start now. If someone has a better idea, let's talk.

10

Cost Shift Realities

We currently spend roughly $2.1 trillion a year on health care in America.[1] That's a huge amount of money. We Americans spend more money on health care than the gross domestic product of 225 countries.[2]

We spend more on health care in total per capita than any other country in the world by a wide margin. Our per capita health care spending in 2004 was $6,280.[3] That compares to Great Britain with $2,546 per capita, Canada with $3,165 per capita, and Germany with $3,043 per capita.[4]

In Canada, England, and Germany, that significantly lower per capita expenditure covers the basic health care needs of every single citizen of those countries. We spend a lot more money on care, yet we still have over forty-five million Americans uninsured at some point every year.[5] We also have an increasing number of Americans who are significantly underinsured.[6] An additional 4 percent of our population believe they have insurance but actually do not.

I'll talk more directly about the uninsured in the next chapter of this book. Before covering that issue, I thought it might be useful to take a quick look at where the revenue actually comes from that pays for the care received now by all of those uninsured Americans.

Uninsured Americans Receive Care

Uninsured Americans do in fact receive care. That care often comes much later in the progression of a disease than it should and it often happens in less-than-optimal care sites (like emergency rooms), but care does happen for uninsured people.[7] The obvious financial problem is that the uninsured people too often simply can't pay for that care. Many people who are uninsured can easily be financially ruined by a single episode of needed care. People's economic lives are damaged and—to add one more complication—the caregivers themselves end up with customers who simply can't pay for the services they have received. Bad debt and bad credit ratings both result.

Some levels of care for uninsured people are legally required. A lot of people do not know that to be true. The law is pretty clear, however, that if someone shows up sick at a hospital, the hospital must provide care, whether or not the person is insured and whether or not the person can pay.[8] So the uninsured do get care, but, as noted earlier, it tends to be expensive care delivered in the wrong place too much of the time.

So is health care somehow magically free to our communities or to society overall if the uninsured patients don't pay for it? Not at all. The cost of providing care for the uninsured has to be met from some revenue source, so that cost is generally shifted to other payers. Someone does, in the end, pay for health care. The question that we all need to understand is, Which other payers actively absorb the burden of that cost shift? That's actually a very important question to understand, because the payers who actually absorb the cost shift America faces today from the uninsured have a real incentive to get out from under that cost shift. Those payers have an equally important incentive not to be the future victims of an even larger cost shift tomorrow, as the number of underinsured and uninsured Americans continues to grow.

Who Pays for the Cost Shift Today?

Since we are not a single payer, government-run health insurance country, we Americans pay for our health care now from multiple sources. Individuals pay. Employers who purchase health benefits for their employees pay. Various charities pay. But the number one source of health care dollars in America is the government. Health care is a huge portion of the total operating budgets of each level in the U.S. government, and those governmental dollars that go to health care all come originally from the taxpayer.

Government

Of the $2 trillion spent annually on health care in America, $420 billion comes from our Medicare programs and over $320 billion comes from our Medicaid programs.[9] Roughly $32 billion comes from our Veteran's Administration (VA) programs,[10] and $2.2 billion comes from our programs to provide health care to Native Americans.[11]

Those programs add up to a total of $774.2 billion—or more than 38 percent of our total American health care dollars. But that is not the total government expenditure for health care. There's another huge piece of the health care budget that also originates from our tax dollars. That other huge piece is money spent to buy health care coverage for government employees and their families. We have a lot of government employees in this country, including the federal government, state government, county government, city, town, and village government, and our various public schools. All told, roughly twenty million Americans get a paycheck from the government.[12] If we assume an average per capita health care premium cost for these employees of $6,000 per year, that adds another $120 billion to the tax dollars spent on American health care, bringing the tax paid total to roughly 44 percent of the total health care spent.

Individuals

So who else pays for health care in America? About one third of the total payment comes from people paying for some portion of their own health care, including their portion of employer-sponsored health insurance premiums.[13] A large percentage of those dollars are spent on types of care not covered by insurance, like nonprescription drugs, dental and nursing home care, medical products, and alternative forms of care. Those "self-pay" dollars typically are not spent in hospitals, clinics, or emergency rooms.

Employers

Finally, 26 percent of the total money spent—or roughly $500 billion—comes from monies paid by the employers who purchase health care coverage for their current and retired employees and their employees' dependents.[14] The $500 billion spent by employers in America is not the biggest piece of the total health care budget, but it looms very large in our national health care economy for two reasons.

One is because, on a pure head count basis, employers cover more actual people than the rest of the payers put together. More than 155 million Americans receive their health coverage from an employer, either their own or that of a family member.[15] The other reason that the payers loom large in funding health care is that two thirds of the uncompensated costs of caring for the uninsured get shifted by care providers to those employers.[16] In other words, employers fund coverage for the largest percentage of our population, and employers fund the lion's share of uncompensated care in America. Figure 10.1 depicts this cost distribution across private and public payers.

Employers in America pay a relatively high amount for health care compared to other countries in the world. Right now, roughly $1,525 of employee and retiree health care cost in an American-

Figure 10.1. Sources of Health Care Funding.

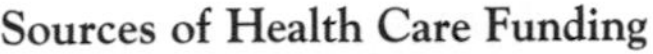

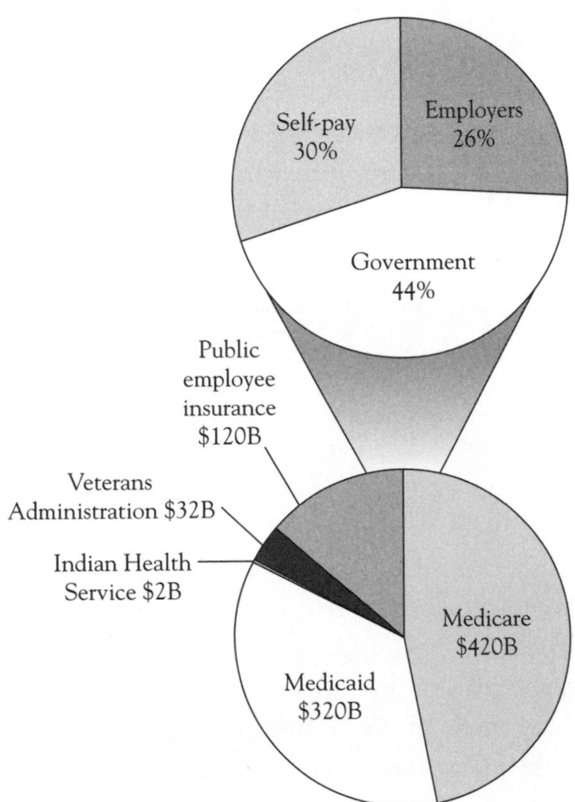

built car has no counterpart in a car built in Japan.[17] See Figure 10.2. As noted earlier, GM spends more money on retiree health care alone than it does on steel.[18] Starbucks spends more on health care than it does on coffee.[19]

American employers currently spend on average more than $4,500 per employee per year to buy health care coverage; employees pay on average $2,000 a year for this coverage.[20] I pointed out earlier that over forty-five million people can be uninsured at some point each

Figure 10.2. Hidden Costs of Health Care in the Price of a $15,000 Car.

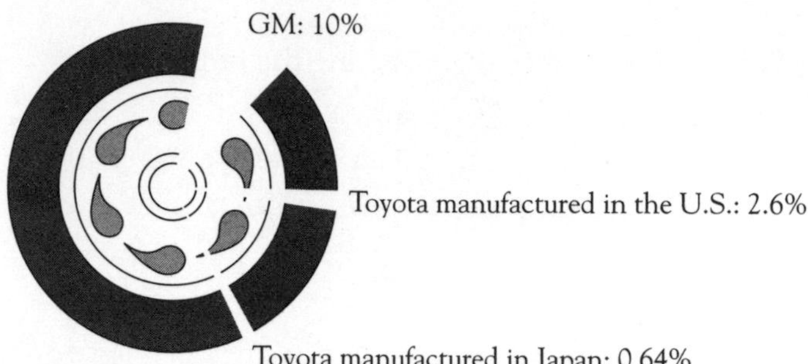

Source: R. French, "GM, Nation Losing Out to Health Care." *Salt Lake Tribune*, Oct. 28, 2006.

year. Those uninsured people pay many of their own health care bills, but a large percentage of those bills are simply not paid.

When the uninsured who are ill and need care can't pay for their hospital or their physician, the uncompensated caregiver simply shifts the cost of that care to the other available payers, to the extent possible. Some cost shift is historically absorbed by federal government subsidies, and some counties and cities also partially subsidize some of that care,[21] but the bulk of the costs of uninsured care gets shifted to the private purchasers of insurance.

Cost Shifting: A Necessary Evil

Cost shifting is not an evil deed—it's a necessary evil. Free care is not cost-free care. Hospitals have real expenses. They pay for supplies, electricity, buildings, and equipment. Hospitals hire nurses, technicians, cleaning crews, and many caregivers and health care professionals. Hospitals have a very legitimate need to meet payroll for their employees who take care of uninsured people, so hospitals shift the cost of those payrolls to their other payers.

How do hospitals shift costs? They simply increase the fees they charge to their insured patients. Hospitals know that the insured patient will pay their bills, so the cost shift is simply added to those patients' bills.

So why do employers end up bearing the brunt of the cost shift? Because the employers then pay those hospital bills through the coverage they provide to their employees. Employers are the only economic "soft touch" in the American universe of payers. Look again at Figure 10.1. Not everyone accepts a cost shift. Medicare and Medicaid do not allow a cost shift to them. The VA and Indian Health Services do not allow a cost shift either. The people who pay for their own health care are not buying that care primarily from hospitals or other providers who care for the uninsured. So, as shown in Figure 10.3, almost the entire impact of the cost shift now falls on the private employers, who pay only $500 billion of the $2 trillion in total health care spending. That is obviously a disproportionate share of expense being shifted to private employers. It adds directly to the cost of private health care coverage.

As the number of uninsured persons grows, that cost shift number is also growing. The impact of shifting these costs to private coverage is now an extra $922 for family insurance and $341 for individual insurance paid by employers. In 2005, more than $43 billion in health care was provided to people without adequate insurance. Of

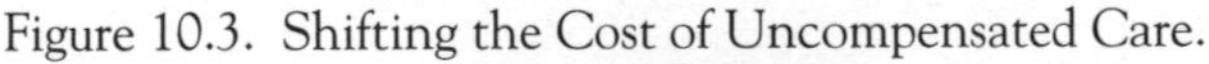
Figure 10.3. Shifting the Cost of Uncompensated Care.

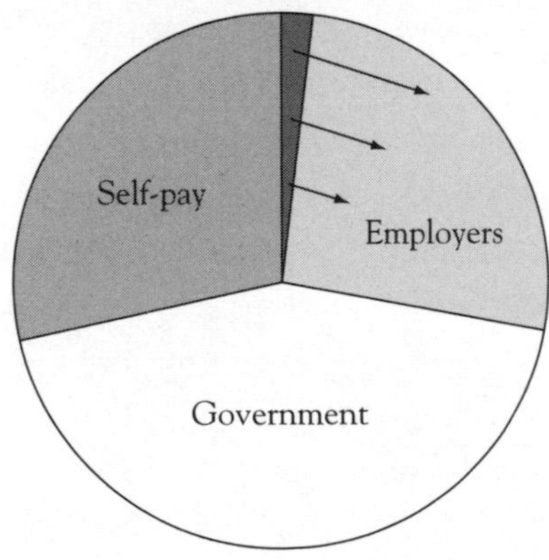

this, $29 billion was financed by higher insurance premiums.[22] That's worth repeating: cost shifts are creating an extra burden of $922 per year per employee, and that number may go over $1,000 by the end of 2007.[23]

Keep that cost shift number in mind as you read the next chapter relative to the funding needed to provide coverage to uninsured Americans. If we put the right universal coverage program in place, we should be able to fund coverage for the uninsured by spending less money for the uninsured than we currently shift to the private employers—with better, more accessible, and more cost-efficient care provided to the uninsured.

So how can we accomplish that goal? That topic is the subject of the next chapter. I believe it can be done, and now is the time to do it. The same factors that will enable better care for the insured—a common provider number, an electronic database for care performance, etc.—can all be directly applied to uninsured Americans as soon as coverage is universal.

In the meantime, the cost shift to the private marketplace will continue to grow, and the uninsured will continue to get inefficient and inadequate care. We can do a lot better. Frankly, we can't afford not to. The cost shift, all by itself, should compel us to act.

11

Universal Coverage Now!

We really cannot achieve total health care reform in America until we have health care coverage for every American. We can't create a database about health care performance that works at the levels we really want while over forty-five million uninsured Americans do not have their care in that database. We can't provide the full continuity of care that we should provide to each American over time as long as large numbers of Americans slip in and out of health care coverage and the care delivery database on an irregular basis. If we really want systematic care improvement in this country, then everyone needs affordable access to systematic care. That will not happen until we achieve universal coverage. This is not, I believe, an impossible dream.

Every other industrialized country in the world offers universal health care coverage to all of their citizens. Every person in England, France, Japan, and Singapore has a pretty complete set of health care benefits mandated by the government of his or her country.

The exact form of universal coverage varies quite a bit from country to country. No two programs are alike. Some countries give vouchers to everyone, and people then use the vouchers to buy coverage from competing private health plans. Others require their citizens to buy coverage directly from the local competing plans. Some countries have a pure single payer approach to health insurance, but allow the actual front-line caregivers to be separate and independent businesses. Others actually employ the caregivers, own the clinics and hospitals, and run every single health care expense through the direct government budget process and cash flow.

The range of variations in universal coverage programs and care delivery is fascinating. Some universal coverage systems own the hospitals but allow the doctors to set up independent physician practices. The physicians in those countries bill the government for patient care. Other models put the physicians on salary. Yet others pay fees. Some pay caregivers on a per capita basis per patient, and a doctor's pay level depends on the size of the "panel of patients" who sign up for that physician's care. Some countries require physicians to work directly for the government, but then allow those same physicians to also have a nongovernment private practice to treat private patients on their days off.

I once helped start a health plan in a European country where the doctors worked primarily for the government, but were available in a different office for a half a day a week to treat private fee-for-service or HMO clients. Nurses could work in those private, independent clinics five days a week. Doctors could work there only a half day a week. So a lot of the care continuity in those clinics depended on the nurses, not the half-day-a-week doctors. The economic model was pretty simple. The doctors received a monthly salary from the government for the patients seen in government clinics and then charged cash fees for the care given to their private patients. That kind of private-public mixture of care systems and care sites happens in quite a few countries. Primary care doctors employed by the National Health Service in England can make up to 10 percent of their income from private practice.[1]

The key point I've learned in looking at a number of universal coverage programs is that no two are alike.

Health Care Solidarity as a Core Value

The specific models used for universal coverage differ widely from country to country. What does not differ at all, however, is the fact that in each of those industrialized countries, coverage truly is universal. Every citizen is covered. In just about all settings, most, if not all, resident noncitizens are also covered. People do not ever worry about being uninsured in some of those countries because they actually couldn't be uninsured, even if they wanted to be. In other countries, where each individual is mandated to purchase his or her own coverage, the coverage is guaranteed and the costs are subsidized for low-income people.

So who pays for universal coverage in those industrialized countries? For low-income people, the answer is the same in all countries. The taxpayers. There are a number of private health insurance products that supplement the government program in some countries, and people are allowed to make more expensive care system choices by paying more money in other countries, but basically in every country the foundational and universal coverage program for low-income people is a direct expense paid by a governmental budget, using taxpayer money. And in a number of countries, the government program provides coverage directly to all citizens. The Scandinavian countries, for example, look a lot like the Canadian system, except for a very nice feature that creates local vertically integrated care systems by township or country. Those local vertically integrated country plans receive budgets and look very much like Kaiser Permanente care units!

With universal coverage programs in place, the various budget and cost issues relating to health care are often the topic of heated public debate in these countries. People debate in very public settings about whether or not a specific community needs an expensive new hospital—or whether the local government hospital needs an additional CT scanner or a new surgery unit.

Open and public debates about exactly how to spend limited health care money are common in countries with universal coverage. But no one debates whether or not any individual resident should or should not be insured. Insurance is a given—a fact of life. The form of insurance varies, but the existence of coverage for everyone is a universal truth. It's a universal expectation—an entitlement of citizenship. The term *solidarity* is heard in health care discussions in many countries. Solidarity in that social context basically means we are all in this health world together. No one should be left behind. No one should be disadvantaged. Everyone should have equal access to basic care. It's a strongly held societal value across Europe. And in the industrialized countries with relatively well-funded universal coverage systems, that belief in solidarity is in fact the basic guideline for developing and operating those systems.

By contrast, even though we Americans spend more money on health care than any other nation in the world by a wide margin, coverage here is absolutely not universal and it is certainly neither an entitlement or a requirement. Solidarity is not a public value written into American law. Depending on whose figures you use, more than forty-five million Americans are uninsured for at least part of each year and of these, roughly twenty million Americans are almost permanently uninsured.[2] Why is that a problem? Far too many people in this country do not get the care they need, in the most appropriate setting for that care, at the best time to receive that care, simply because those people are uninsured. We are less healthy as a society because a very large percentage of our population has no health coverage.

Cost Shift Could Pay for Universal Care

As pointed out in Chapter Ten, the uninsured in the United States do not go entirely without care. Far from it. People who are uninsured do receive certain levels of care in America. Americans also believe that society should guarantee some level of health. We share that societal value with other people around the world.

In America, however, we don't insert the requirement that care be available into the health care equation until someone is in serious trouble. We believe no one should die from a lack of medical help. So we have laws mandating that emergency rooms and hospitals accept anyone who is very sick and comes to their doors.[3] A form of partial universal coverage in America ends up happening badly, in the form of mandatory available emergency and hospital care. Very often, however, as I noted earlier the uninsured people receiving care do not have the ability to pay for that care. Care received by the uninsured and not paid for constitutes a significant cost burden on almost all caregivers—to the point that credible and reputable projections show a cost shift from the uninsured to the insured population of roughly $29 billion a year.[4]

So who pays for that "uncompensated" care? As we discussed in the previous chapter, providers do not "eat" the cost of care to the uninsured—they shift that cost to other payers.

Specifically, providers of care shift most of the cost of caring for uninsured patients to their insured patients. How is that done? By simply raising the fees charged to those insured patients—to the point where the cost of private health insurance in America is nearly 9 percent higher than it would be if everyone in the United States had health care.[5] That currently equals roughly $1,100 per employee per year for family coverage in California.[6] In other words, without the current cost shift, the price of family insurance premiums in California could be $1,100 lower right now.

As you will read later in this chapter, that's almost exactly how much money we actually would need to provide universal coverage to all of our citizens. It's pretty easy to run numbers showing that if that same $1,100 were spent much more appropriately, the total cost of providing coverage to the uninsured could be accomplished without adding any real new money to the total health care economy. And the cost shift to employers and privately insured people could be ended.

That's one of the great ironies and challenges of the American health care economy. We already spend enough money on everyone to cover everyone—we just don't spend it in ways that will directly increase the breadth of coverage to the point where everyone is actually covered. We have enough money to pay for solidarity in American health care. We just don't have the infrastructure in place to achieve it.

The proposal shown later in this chapter will explain a way that we could raise enough money to cover all of the uninsured and do it in a way that will not only end the current cost shift, but also create a more effective, accountable, and results-focused total health care system.

Racial and Ethnic Disparities in Coverage and Care

Before going to the specific elements of that universal coverage proposal, I'd like to make a couple of other points about the nature of the total cost and health status burden this country faces by not having universal health care coverage in place. I believe that whenever we look at the issue of the uninsured without looking at these key data points and societal realities, we are sidestepping an important set of moral, ethical, and social issues that we really ought to have the honesty and courage to address as a society. So what are these issues? Prejudice, discrimination, and disparity. Multiple studies have shown that disparities in both health coverage and health care exist in this country relative to ethnic and racial differences in both health status and care patterns that occur every day in our current nonsystem of care. The Institute of Medicine's report *Unequal Treatment: Confronting Racial and Ethnic Disparities in Health Care* is a comprehensive introduction to the topic.[7] The Commonwealth Fund has written several excellent reports on that topic as well.[8]

As noted earlier, asthma is growing at epidemic proportions for all of our children. African American children face by far the heaviest asthma burden and receive by far the lowest level of asthma care. The death rate from asthma for African American children is four times higher than the death rate for white children.[9] Look at Exhibits 11.1, 11.2, 11.3, and 11.4 to get a sense of the extent of the disparities children and adults experience in health care based on their ethnicity. We, as caring Americans, should find those facts unconscionable. A country committed to health care equity for all of its citizens should be totally unaccepting of numbers showing that any portion of our children routinely are deprived of health or care by an unaccountable and unavailable health care nonsystem. We should be even more unaccepting when those unnecessary deprivations are directly linked to race, ethnicity, and culture.

Exhibits 11.1, 11.2, 11.3, and 11.4 show similar health care disparity numbers for a multitude of other issues. For example, the death rate from heart disease for African American women is 36 percent higher than the death rate for white women.[10] The level of appropriate diabetic care for African American men and women lags behind performance levels for white Americans.[11]

Why do I mention those facts in a chapter on universal coverage? Because, to no one's surprise, there is a direct correlation between health insurance coverage and health care—and the rate of being uninsured is also nearly double for African Americans compared to white Americans.[12] Minority Americans make up roughly one-third of our total population but well over half of our uninsured population.[13] In California, 75 percent of the uninsured are minority groups.[14]

Those numbers make both health care delivery and health care coverage a very direct racial and ethnic equity issue. The American distribution of care, coverage, and health is a very long way from solidarity.

We've come a long way on most of our other major racial equity issues in America. We now have extensive laws about equal opportunity on the job. We have ended almost all discrimination relative to voting rights. Over the past fifty years, we Americans have made major progress in multiple areas relative to racial and ethnic discrimination. That is excellent news. We should be proud of that progress in those key areas relating to the legal status of all Americans. But we definitely have not made equal progress on health status. The numbers I've just cited prove that the area where we still

Exhibit 11.1. Disparities in Health Care Services.

- A study of the relationship between quality and racial disparity among 151 Medicare health plans found that performance on four outcome measures (blood glucose control for enrollees with diabetes, cholesterol control for enrollees with diabetes or heart disease, and blood pressure control) was lower for black enrollees than for white ones by 7 to 14 percent.[1]
- Blacks, Asians, and Hispanics are significantly less likely than whites to receive care at hospitals with more experience at performing certain complex surgical procedures.[2]
- Physicians are less likely to prescribe opioid pain medications to black emergency room patients than either Latinos or whites.[3]
- Black, Hispanic, and Asian/Pacific Islander health care–eligible veterans are half as likely to report ambulatory care use than are white veterans.[4]

[1]A. N. Trivedi, A. M. Zaslavsky, E. C. Schneider, and J. Z. Ayanian. "Relationship Between Quality of Care and Racial Disparities in Medicare Health Plans." *Journal of the American Medical Association*, 2006, *296*(16), 1998–2004.

[2]J. H. Liu and others. "Disparities in the Utilization of High-Volume Hospitals for Complex Surgery." *Journal of the American Medical Association*, 2006, *296*(16), 2026–2027.

[3]J. H. Tamayo-Sarver, S. W. Hinze, R. K. Cydulka, and D. W. Baker. "Racial and Ethnic Disparities in Emergency Department Analgesic Prescription." *American Journal of Public Health*, 2003, 93(12), 2067–2073.

[4]D. L. Washington and others. "Racial/Ethnic Variations in Veterans' Ambulatory Care Use." *American Journal of Public Health*, 2005, 95(12), 2231–2237.

fail most miserably in ending racial and ethnic disparities is in health care. We still have huge and undeniable inequities relative to who has health care coverage, and we have equivalently huge and undeniable inequities and inequalities relative to the actual delivery of care. Those numbers should be on the policy debate table every single day.

If we looked at no issue other than racial and ethnic disparities in American health care, our leadership from all parties and all

Exhibit 11.2. Disparities in Cancer Incidence and Care.

- African Americans are more likely to be diagnosed with and die of colorectal cancer than white patients.[1]
- African American men are more likely to develop and die from oral and pharyngeal cancer.[2]
- Hispanic and African American men with prostate cancer received less medical monitoring than did white men.[3]
- Black and Hispanic women are less likely to be diagnosed with early-stage breast cancer than are white women.[4] Black American women are 19 percent more likely than white women to die of breast cancer, and they are half as likely as white women to receive recommended postsurgical drug treatment for breast cancer.

[1] B. N. Polite, J. J. Dignam, and O. I. Olopade. "Colorectal Cancer Model of Health Disparities: Understanding Mortality Differences in Minority Populations." *Journal of Clinical Oncology*, 2006, *24*(14), 2179–2187.

[2] A. McLean and others. "Disparities in Oral and Pharyngeal Cancer Incidence and Mortality Among Wisconsin Residents, 1999-2002." *Wisconsin Medical Journal*, 2006, *105*(6), 32–35.

[3] V. L. Shavers and others. "Race/Ethnicity and the Intensity of Medical Monitoring While Under 'Watchful Waiting' for Prostate Cancer." *Medical Care*, 2004, *42*(3), 239–250.

[4] P. M. Lantz and others. "The Influence of Race, Ethnicity, and Individual Socioeconomic Factors on Breast Cancer Stage at Diagnosis." *American Journal of Public Health*, 2006, 96(12), 2173–2178.

[5] HealthDay News. "Black Women More Likely to Die of Breast Cancer." Mar. 21, 2006.

community groups should be moving this country down the path to an American form of universal coverage as quickly as we can. We should not be able as a nation to maintain a sense of clean conscience and then simply not deal with those major ethnic and racial disparity issues relative to people being uninsured—particularly when we can now accomplish those goals for the first time in the context of a total health care reform agenda that could improve the quality and efficiency of care for everyone while extending coverage

Exhibit 11.3. Disparities in Chronic Conditions.

- African Americans have the highest overall coronary artery disease mortality rate and the highest out-of-hospital coronary death rate of any ethnic group in the United States.[1]
- Blacks and Hispanics are three to four times more likely to be hospitalized for diabetes with long-term complications, for diabetes-related foot amputations, and for high blood pressure than are whites.
- Blacks have the highest rates of preventable hospital admissions for conditions such as congestive heart failure, asthma, perforated appendicitis, and dehydration.[2]
- African American women have the highest mortality rate for asthma of all groups, more than 2.5 times higher than white women.[3]
- Aging non-Hispanic blacks and Hispanics have higher risk for severe pain than do non-Hispanic whites.[4]
- Black and Hispanic stroke survivors report a lower health-related quality of life than do white stroke survivors.[5]
- Rates of blindness from diabetes are half as high for whites as for the rest of the population.[6]
- Among those with need, white adults are more likely than Hispanic or African American adults to receive active alcoholism, drug abuse, or mental health treatment.[7]
- Hispanics are less likely to receive smoking cessation advice from physicians than are non-Hispanic blacks, non-Hispanic whites, and other non-Hispanic patients.[8]

[1] L. T. Clark. "Issues in Minority Health: Atherosclerosis and Coronary Heart Disease in African Americans." *Medical Clinics of North America,* 2005, 89(5), 977–1001.

[2] J. H. Price. "Diabetic Blacks, Hispanics Face More Hospitalizations." *Washington Times*, Aug. 3, 2006.

[3] Asthma and Allergy Foundation of America. "Asthma Facts and Figures." http://www.aafa.org/display.cfm?id=8&sub=42#disp.

Exhibit 11.3. Disparities in Chronic Conditions, Cont'd.

[4]C. C. Reyes-Gibby and others. "Pain in Aging Community-Dwelling Adults in the United States: Non-Hispanic Whites, Non-Hispanic Blacks, and Hispanics." *Journal of Pain*, 2007, 8(1), 75–84.

[5]J. Xie and others. "Impact of Stroke on Health-Related Quality of Life in the Noninstitutionalized Population in the United States." *Stroke*, 2006, 37(10), 2567–2572.

[6]Agency for Healthcare Research and Quality. "Fact Sheet: Diabetes Disparities Among Racial and Ethnic Minorities." Nov. 2001.

[7]K. Wells, R. Klap, A. Koike, and C. Sherbourne. "Ethnic Disparities in Unmet Need for Alcoholism, Drug Abuse, and Mental Health Care." *American Journal of Psychiatry*, 2001, *158*(12), 2027–2032.

[8]C. Lopez-Quintero, R. M. Crum, and Y. D. Neumark. "Racial/Ethnic Disparities in Report of Physician-Provided Smoking Cessation Advice: Analysis of the 2000 National Health Interview Survey." *American Journal of Public Health*, 2006, 96(12), 2235–2239.

to all Americans. A major part of the reform agenda we need in America is based on finally having a database that lets us track care delivery and improve care performance. That agenda cannot reach full levels of success while more than forty-five million people are not included in it. We need everyone covered so we can make the infrastructure completely accountable.

Finding a Universal Coverage Model

The American approach to universal health coverage needs to be an American model. As I noted earlier, universal coverage in France doesn't look like at all universal coverage in Germany or the United Kingdom. Each county has found its own path to providing both coverage and care to all of its citizens. For a snapshot of the differences, see Table 11.1. We couldn't adopt the British system if we wanted to—with the U.S. government taking over direct ownership of all the hospitals and then funding each of the doctors in this

Exhibit 11.4. Disparities for Children and Teens.

- In terms of mortality rates for white infants, the United States ranks thirty-fifth among nations. In terms of mortality rates for black infants, the United States ranks eighty-fourth.[1]
- Among urban children with asthma, Latinos are five times more likely and African Americans are twice as likely to use urgent care (emergency room and hospital care).[2] Latino and black children have worse asthma status and are three to ten times less likely to use preventive medications than white children.[3]
- Hispanic and African American teens are more likely than their white peers to sustain a serious work-related injury, despite job similarities.[4]
- Black and Hispanic children have a higher death rate after congenital heart surgery than do white children.[5]

[1]Central Intelligence Agency. "The World Factbook: Rank Order—Infant Mortality Rate." Nov. 2006; Department of Health and Human Services. "Fact Sheet: Preventing Infant Mortality." Jan. 2006.

[2]J. A. Stingone and L. Claudio. "Disparities in the Use of Urgent Health Care Services Among Asthmatic Children." *Annals of Allergy, Asthma, and Immunology*, 2006, 97(2), 244–250.

[3]J. A. Finkelstein and others. "Quality of Care for Preschool Children with Asthma: The Role of Social Factors and Practice." *Pediatrics*, 1995, 95, 389–394.

[4]K. M. Zierold and H. A. Anderson. "Racial and Ethnic Disparities in Work-Related Injuries Among Teenagers." *Journal of Adolescent Health*, 2006, 39(3), 422–426.

[5]O. J. Benavidez, K. Gauvreau, and K. J. Jenkins. "Racial and Ethnic Disparities in Mortality Following Congenital Heart Surgery." *Pediatric Cardiology*, 2006, 37(3), 321–328.

country directly. We might find the German system easier to use, with each citizen selecting his or her own health plan (or "Sickness Fund") from a competing marketplace of over three hundred private funds.[15] Citizens are required to maintain health insurance through contributions to the fund of their choice, which then provides any needed care. Citizens can pay more or less money out of pocket, depending on which sickness fund they select.

Table 11.1. Germany, Canada, and the United Kingdom Health Systems: A Brief Comparison.

	Germany	Canada	United Kingdom
Care system	Social insurance relying on 300 statutory sickness funds	National health insurance	National Health Service
Payment source	Employers and employees share premium costs set as percentage of income	Federal and provincial funds	Local authorities administer national and local funds
Physician payment	Sickness funds pay physicians on fee-for-service basis through fee-setting regional medical associations	Provincial governments set fee schedules; physicians bill government directly	General practitioners (GPs) are self-employed; payment from local trust is based on capitation, fixed allowances, and quality points.
Hospital ownership	Diverse: roughly 50% publicly owned, 40% private nonprofit, and 10% private for profit	Largely private nonprofit with annual global operating budget from province	Overwhelmingly publicly owned; <5% of hospital beds are privately owned.
Private insurance	10% of population opts out of state system	By law, limited to care not available through public system	11% of population owns "queue-jumping" private insurance
Primary care availability	Same-day appointments	Primary care wait times of increasing concern	NHS met target of <48-hour wait for GP appointments
Specialty care availability	No referral needed; widely available	Primary care physicians act as gatekeepers. Overall median wait: 3 days for urgent cases; 5 to 6 weeks for elective cases.	GPs act as gatekeepers. Wait times for specialty care are significant (e.g., 56 to 168 days for inpatient cardiac surgery).

Sources: R. S. Galvin. "Physician Payment in Canada, Germany, and the United States." *Physician Executive*, May-June 1993; Civitas. "Health Care in Germany." 2005; Civitas. "Background Briefing: The Canadian Health Care System." 2005; British Columbia Medical Association. "Specialty Care in BC: A System in Distress." June 2004; College of Family Physicians of Canada. "Media Backgrounder." News release, Nov. 2, 2006; King's Fund. "NHS Waiting Times." News release, Jan. 4, 2005; World Health Organization. "Highlights on Health, United Kingdom 2004." Feb. 2006; National Health Service. "Waiting Times." http://www.nhs.uk/England/AboutTheNHS/WaitingTimes/Default.cmsx.

The German model was actually invented by Otto von Bismarck in 1883, when he was chancellor of Germany. No one can argue that it hasn't withstood the test of time, even though it is severely financially challenged today in many ways. Again, transplanting the German model to the United States might have its advocates, but it's not a perfect fit for our culture and it doesn't optimize use of some of the best parts of our medical economy and infrastructure.

We need an American model. We need a model that mixes features involving government funding for some patients and private funding for others.

America's Employer-Based Model

We also need, as I have said repeatedly in this book, an American model that deliberately involves employers as an enlightened, innovative, and demanding purchasing agent for coverage and care. We need smart buyers in health care. Employers can play that role. Some people in the United States assume that other countries who have universal coverage for their citizens simply and completely exclude private employers from any role in paying for or selecting health coverage. Some do. But others involve employers very directly and extensively. Multiple options exist.

Following a European universal coverage model would not preclude having a significant role in our American model for employer-based coverage. In several European countries, there is often a direct link between each person's employer and the specific health care coverage mechanism used by the employee. In some countries, the employers collect a payroll tax and then help select health plans for their employees. In other countries, the employers don't buy the basic universal coverage, but they do purchase supplemental plans that provide additional layers of health insurance for their employees—over and above the universal health coverage paid for by the government.

In the United Kingdom, for example, many employers contract with BUPA (British United Provident Association) or its competitors to provide extra levels of health insurance coverage. Why would anyone in Britain buy that additional coverage? Convenience and access. The NHS does a great job of providing primary care, but there have been some long waiting times for specialty care in some areas of the country. BUPA offers insurance plans that allow sick people who don't want to wait in the sometimes long lines required for certain specialty services in the National Health Insurance program to "queue-jump" and get their treatments or surgeries quite a bit faster from the private caregiver marketplace in Britain. Those private "wrap-around" plans are a fairly popular option. Roughly six and a half million people in England have purchased that kind of "queue-jump" supplemental insurance, usually through their employers.[16] Some labor unions also negotiate BUPA coverage for their members. In Ireland, with a very similar government basic health system model, roughly two million people buy queue-jump supplemental plans from Vhi Healthcare, Vivas Healthcare, or BUPA Ireland.[17]

BUPA, by the way, also owns and runs a network of private hospitals in Britain to facilitate that whole concept of giving quicker access to certain levels of care for BUPA patients. The private hospitals also claim to offer a more competitive service level to their members.

In any case, employers in many universal health care countries either buy BUPA-like coverage for their workers or contract for basic coverage as an agent for the government. I mention those points in this book because it's important for people thinking about universal coverage to know that every other country that has already achieved that goal has done so after going through a creative design process that fits their own situation, their own citizenry, and their own goals. I believe we need to go through a similar America-specific process, evolving a universal coverage approach that fits our own situation and goals—one that meets the needs of our citizens for choice, quality, efficiency, affordability, accessibility, and continuity—enhancing care without undermining key elements of our American expectations about care.

The Canadian Model: Budget Control

To the extent that Americans do suggest that we should consider imparting another country's solution to our nation, the plan I hear mentioned most often is Canada. "Why can't we just use the Canadian system?" people ask. "They have universal coverage and spend a lot less money than we do in the process." Why can't we clone Canada?

Let me discuss that model briefly. Everyone in Canada has coverage. That is true. That's definitely a very good thing. That coverage is universal, with most local provincial governments as the only legal insurers. Each plan is funded by each province through its own tax base. Local taxes, local care. That approach could work in the United States—although we would need to go through a challenging period of transition to figure out how to set up a tax base in each state sufficient to buy coverage for everyone. We might want to figure out how not to lose all of the dollars now spent on health care from various nongovernmental sources. Those would be complicated and complex discussions, but they would not be the most challenging aspects of the Canadian system relative to our country. The most challenging aspect would be our need to have the government of each of our states take full financial control and provincial ownership of what are now, in this country, private hospitals and private care delivery programs. Hospitals in Canada function basically as public-funded branches of the government, not private economic entities.

In Canada, the government actually dictates the annual hospital revenue levels for each hospital, and the government controls the costs of Canadian health care largely by controlling both hospital capacity and annual hospital budgets. The government also sets local budgets for physician spending. The government invests disproportionately in primary care, so primary care in Canada is pretty much universally available—although concerns have been expressed recently about primary care wait times.[18] Specialty care is a bit more limited in Canada, deliberately receiving a lower level of investments. Hospital availability and expenses are tightly controlled by the simple fact that the government directly controls the revenue streams of all hospitals. Each hospital has a budget set by the government. When those budgets run out, care tends to change significantly.

In Canada, in November or December, if a local hospital runs out of budget money for the year, in many cases the hospital simply puts non-emergency treatment on hold for a couple of months until a new budget period begins. Exceeding those annual individual hospital budgets is often not allowed except for emergencies. That level of direct control over hospital expenses and availability is actually a very workable model if you really want to control costs. It seems to fit the Canadian culture. It creates real solidarity, because everyone is in the same boat. But it's not clear that most Americans would tolerate delaying non-emergency surgeries and treatments for a month or two when state-given budgets run out for local hospitals. It's also not clear that Americans would tolerate a solidarity-enhancing law that would make it illegal for any American to buy care directly from a doctor.

Canada does spend less money than we do on health care. Why? Some of the cost savings in Canada result from the government being the only insurer. Canada's administrative costs are often one-third of American administrative costs. But when you do the math, those well-publicized administrative cost savings in Canada account for less than a fifth of the actual cost differences between American care and Canadian care. Much larger portions of those Canadian cost savings result from the provincial governments having direct budget control over each provider of care.

Is America ready for that approach to saving health care dollars?

I suspect that we might be in a few years if we can't make other, more flexible, and more patient-focused care delivery reform models work.

The British System: Rationed Care

One key point to consider in thinking about whether the U.S. government would do as well as the Canadian government serving as a new single payer for health care is to determine whether our government would actually be willing to make the same kinds of difficult cost-based decisions that have given governments in some other single payer countries significantly more control over actual expenditures for care. There is a rationing element inherent in any government-imposed budget relative to care. Governments with fixed budgets can't pay for all possible care, so governments on budgets make decisions about how much care will be available. That's just common sense. And basic arithmetic.

Governments in a number of those other universal coverage countries naturally end up making very conscious decisions in their annual budgeting processes to ration access to some levels and types of care. Rationing decisions are made openly, sometimes by formula. The British National Institute for Clinical Excellence (NICE) system, for example, sets a range of £25,000 to £35,000 for "one good year of life." As I write this, that would be equivalent to about $47,000 to $66,000 in the United States. If a new drug or technology can't deliver at least one good and healthy year of life for each £30,000 spent, the British government generally does not allow that drug, procedure, or technology into the National Health Service (NHS) system.[19]

That NICE process does not now exist at any level in the United States. It is part of the accepted "solidarity" culture of Great Britain. The concept of solidarity allows for the public acceptance of NICE. Why? Because everyone is subject to the same set of rules when it comes to access to the government-rationed care. Rationing is done in an absolutely evenhanded way. That's the explicit approach. The open approach. The NICE approach.

Some of the other care-rationing processes that governments use are not equally explicit. For example, the British government also seems to consciously build too few heart hospitals and hire too few heart surgeons for all possible and potential heart surgeries. Why is that a form of rationing? The absence of the new heart hospital means that certain heart patients will not get their surgeries. The open and public debate might be about the cost of the hospital to the local taxpayer. The functional, implicit result of that decision will be about the real-world availability or nonavailability of transplants to local heart patients.

But those discussions are not as explicit and the outcomes are not as clear. In the United States, we build enough capacity for all our insured heart patients. Why? Because each insured American patient comes with a built-in cash flow and a solid fee-for-service payment guarantee. Patients are revenue in the United States. In Britain, each heart patient is an expense, and these patients come to British hospitals with no revenue and no potential to earn a margin. So hospital building decisions are looked at very differently in each country.

Medicare for All: Would the U.S. Government Ration Care?

When you look at how each country makes its budgeting decisions relative to care infrastructure, care technology, and caregiver staffing, it's pretty clear that single payer universal coverage countries all ration in some way relative to the total availability of care. Would our government also ration in some way if we had a single payer system like the Canadian system of universal Medicare? Of course it would.

Our government does that now. Look at the fact that Congress deliberately and very consciously totally rationed drug coverage for

American seniors for nearly forty years and then, when the government finally introduced Medicare Part D coverage (a long overdue decision, by the way), it designed the new drug benefits on a blatantly rationed basis with a deliberate payment hole in the middle of the benefit coverage for quite a few seniors. That benefit hole exists only to save money. It's difficult to administer and hard to explain. But it does save money. Our lawmakers rationed. Give me another explanation for that benefit and I would be delighted to learn it. The jury is in, I am afraid. Rationing happened here. Again. Our Congress rationed care. It happens all the time when the government pays for care.

More directly and much more widely, look back at the decisions made every year by both state and national government to limit both Medicaid coverage and Medicaid eligibility. In each case, to save money, the government rationed. Coverage was extended to fewer people. That is rationing. Benefits are often reduced for Medicaid patients purely as the result of state budget cuts. That is also rationing. The fact that multiple American governmental units who are responsible for health care budgets decide to ration should not be surprising. It's what governments all over the world do when faced with expensive health care choices—whenever costs exceed budgets.

Interestingly, as I noted earlier relative to NICE, those rationing decisions seem to have a relatively high level of political acceptance in many other countries. Why is that true? Because, as one European citizen I talked to told me, "Those cuts affect all of us equally. No one in this country gets a heart transplant. We don't discriminate in the choice of who gets a transplant based on economic status. Solidarity prevails—both for what is available and for what is not available."

In America we don't have that equivalent absolute sense of equality relative to accessibility to care. Solidarity is not an operating principle. Our care availability in America is sometimes influenced quite a bit by our personal economic status. And by our insurance coverage status. Our governmental units ration care. But interestingly, our private markets are built on the exact opposite theory of care as an entitlement for the insured, and our provider reimbursement and infrastructure growth decisions are both built on the availability of insured patients, not the deliberations of elected officials and the availability of county or provincial health budget taxpayers' money.

When elected officials do get involved in funding health care here, however, they just act like elected officials do everywhere in the world. Our prisons actually offer a pretty obvious and recently very well-publicized current example of the practical impact that limited governmental funds tend to have on the health care spending decisions made by our lawmakers.[20] Health care in the prisons is totally a government responsibility. It's a pure single payer system funded by our government. How well is that care funding process going? Not well. Badly, in fact. Health care resources in our prisons are rationed and limited to the point that courts are stepping in to deal with the resulting quality-of-care issues in a number of prison settings.

I'm not suggesting that health care for prisoners and "Medicare for everyone" are equivalent programs. They are not—except to note that when health care costs create a budget crisis for any unit of any level of any government anywhere in the world, the decision-making patterns I've seen are pretty similar. We can't always rely on the leadership of American governmental units, who are often in the middle of fighting a real local and immediate budget crunch to simply make all necessary resources available for health care uses. Rationing happens. The basic fact that we do not have universal coverage in America today proves that rationing in fact happens here. For more than forty-five million uninsured people, our policymakers have rationed care.

Up to now, that rationing has happened in America below the conscious radar screen for most of our insured citizenry. At a more conscious level, polls show that our citizens are very much opposed to health care rationing.

It is, of course, possible that given the rapid explosion in American health care costs, maybe some levels of rationing might begin to find growing support with a significant portion of our population. People might demand some form of rationing if the alternative is completely unaffordable costs of care. That would be a shame. My own sense is that rationing should absolutely not be our lead strategy either for health care reform or for health care cost controls. We have so many completely unused, commonsense, systematic process improvement approaches available to us to cut the cost of care in America by consistently and strategically providing better and more proactive care that, I believe, we should go a long way down that care reengineering path before deciding to use a care rationing approach.

I believe any short-term approach that relies on state or local governments directly or indirectly, explicitly or implicitly, using rationing as a key weapon against health care costs would be a shortsighted and counterproductive strategic agenda. We can do a lot better by focusing our care delivery expertise on helping our highest-cost patients. We can do a lot better by bringing process improvement techniques to health care delivery. We should be able to improve care and still cover everyone at the same time. We should, however, now take the steps necessary to cover everyone. How can that be done?

Universal Coverage Now!

Rather than advocate a U.S. version of the Canadian approach to insurance and the ownership of care, I'd like to suggest an American approach that also gets us fairly quickly to universal coverage. The working title of this proposal is Universal Coverage Now or UCN. This UCN proposal builds in part on our existing Medicaid infrastructure, expands the availability of care, and utilizes employer-based coverage (without a cost shift) as a major purchasing tool for making the marketplace more responsive and affordable.

The goal of this UCN proposal is literally universal coverage.

The goal is to cover everyone. It is not a plan to merely incrementally increase the number of insured persons. It's a plan to insure everyone in America, very quickly. Universal. Coverage. Because it is intended to cover everyone, the plan has several key components. It is not a clone of the Canadian single payer model, with just one insurance mechanism. It's closer to the German or Swiss models, involving a mixture of private market coverage and government-run and -subsidized coverage programs.

- Part A of the UCN proposal sets up universal coverage as a mandated benefit.
- Part B funds it.
- Part C measures how well the program is doing and provides a context for accountability and continuous improvement.
- Part D describes a specific benefit plan design for the uninsured that I believe will make the most sense at this point in our history. The benefit package is the least important part of the proposal, but it's worth discussion.

The UCN plan outlined below includes costs estimates, funding sources, regulatory requirements, needed infrastructure, and specific benefits packages. It recommends roles for all key players—consumers, patients, care providers, health plans, governmental agencies, and political leaders. It's a plan built on practicality, using working pieces that can all function in the real world. It's a plan assembled by folks whose day job is to do functional and operational things, so it should hold together as a workable process of practical interlocking proposals that can in total provide coverage to everyone in this country in an effective, affordable, and sustainable way.

Let's look at each piece of the proposal, one piece at a time. The basic foundation of the plan is for the government to pass a law creating the new legal requirement for everyone to be covered. That is Part A of the plan—achieving universal coverage through an individual mandate.

Part A: Individual Coverage Mandate

To achieve universal coverage, I believe we need to start with an explicit and universal individual mandate—a legal requirement that each American have health insurance. Why set up an individual mandate? Unless we have an individual mandate, some people will choose not to be covered. If some people choose not to be covered, we will never get to universal coverage. Without a mandate, in other words, universal coverage will not happen. There is no voluntary path to universal coverage. The law needs to require that every single person acquire coverage. Where will that coverage for everyone come from? Several sources.

- Higher-income people could buy the coverage directly.
- Working people could receive it from their employers.
- Seniors would continue to receive Medicare.
- Lower-income people would continue to receive Medicaid.
- All others would be enrolled in a special HealthPrime entitlement program outlined in this proposal or enrolled in private insurance, "guaranteed issue" products set up to be financially credible. In either case, everyone must buy coverage.

So how will we know if someone has coverage? That is obviously a key question that needs to be answered. Like every part of the proposal, the approach used was to build off something in our overall process that already exists and already works.

The proposed Universal Coverage Now enrollment process accomplishes that goal by building off a key, in-place, governmental infrastructure we all know and love—our tax collection process. Every year at tax filing time, each taxpayer in America would be required to include written proof of health insurance as part of his or her tax filing. Those Americans who are not required to file would have an incentive to file, because it would be through filing that they would receive their health care benefit.

This filing process would be similar to the process of getting a car license: each person now has to show proof of auto insurance in order to get or renew a car license. Similarly, when filing taxes, you would need to show proof of health insurance. Anyone who has a health plan offered by their employer could simply show proof of that insurance as a document attached to their 1040. People with a personally-purchased private plan could also show proof of that insurance. People receiving insurance through a government program like Medicare would show proof of that insurance. For people who show proof of insurance, the tax filing process would be complete relative to health coverage and nothing else would need to be done.

A High-Deductible Plan for Higher-Income Uninsured People

If a person has no insurance, however, then the annual tax filing would trigger a process to sell coverage directly and immediately to the uninsured person. Anyone making more than 300 percent of the federal poverty level who does not have proof of insurance would be forced to actually purchase a plan directly from the government at that point. The government-issued plan for higher-income people will have a high deductible—both because people with income beyond 300 percent of federal poverty are more likely to have enough money to pay for basic health care costs and because it's important to keep the actual premium level as low as possible whenever we force people to buy their own coverage.

Actuarial estimates are that the government can break even and even make a small profit today by selling a $10,000 deductible plan to those high-income uninsured people for roughly $100 a month. The entire year of coverage would be paid for those uninsured, higher-income Americans in advance at tax time as part of the tax filing.

If the higher-income person then chooses at some point during the year to use the private marketplace to buy private coverage instead of just keeping the government high-deductible plan, part of the year's premium paid at tax time to the government plan would be refunded. The refund level should be set at a point where the government benefits a bit financially. There is no point in the government losing money on those post–tax filing insurance coverage decisions made by the higher-income uninsured.

Obviously, the higher-income people would be very much incented every year to buy their own more desirable coverage from the private market well in advance of tax day. Some private market reforms would be needed to guarantee availability of coverage. But, in order to guarantee universal coverage, anyone who doesn't do that will automatically be insured on that tax filing date for a full year by the government by simply adding the year's premium to their tax bill. Taxes will be in arrears if that year's check doesn't come in with the tax form.

Medicaid for the Lowest-Income Uninsured

What about lower-income people? Lower-income people need subsidized or free coverage. I cowrote a paper for *Health Affairs* magazine recently with two other authors, Jay Crosson and Steve Zatkin, about how to achieve universal coverage for California.[21] You can pull that article up on the Internet at HealthAffairs.org at any time. We wrote about a number of alternative approaches to subsidizing coverage for the lower-income uninsured populations.

What we suggested in that article was that the very lowest-income people should qualify for an expedited enrollment process into Medicaid that could be done using electronic tools. All very low-income Americans—male and female, single and family—should be Medicaid eligible. The tax form can be rewritten slightly to tell people how to best use the basic Medicaid enrollment process, and the tax form itself can give both phone numbers and web sites to link people to robust support systems that can help those with low income enroll in coverage. There are some very nice tools that have been developed to perform these enrollment tasks for current entitlement programs, and those tools are very much underutilized. Various clinics and care sites can and should also have access to those expedited enrollment tools, so that uninsured people can be enrolled at the point of receiving care. We particularly need year-round Medicaid enrollment for our very lowest-income population—both male and female—and we also need that enrollment to be facilitated as part of the tax filing process. For people who don't file taxes, enrollment should be expedited through the various community groups and caregivers who take care of uninsured people, with tax filing facilitated when the coverage renews.

Medicaid right now discriminates in its eligibility rules in favor of families. Not all poor people are eligible. Single people without kids who are poor are excluded, in fact. That distinction should be eliminated. Everyone, male or female, whose income is below the federal poverty level should be covered by Medicaid. Likewise, the existing program to cover children—SCHIP—should be expanded to cover families up to 200 percent or 300 percent of the federal poverty level depending on how much money the government agrees to raise to subsidize coverage. The expansion of Medicaid eligibility in those two areas could cover nearly half of the uninsured population immediately—with particular short-term success in extending coverage to our minority populations, who tend to have disproportionately lower incomes and would therefore be eligible for both Medicaid and SCHIP in large numbers much more quickly.

For people who are not Medicaid-eligible but are at less than 200 percent of the federal poverty level and who do not have any health coverage from their employer, the UCN proposal is that coverage for that population also be free—subsidized entirely by the government. So where would coverage for those people come from? People over the federal poverty level but below 200 percent of the poverty level—or between 200 and 300 percent of poverty level—should be able to obtain fully or partially subsidized coverage from a special new program called HealthPrime that uses the Medicaid infrastructure for its administration and also makes private health plans and IVs available as care delivery options.

HealthPrime for All Other Uninsured People

Anyone in that low-income level who does not have other coverage should be granted coverage in a brand new HealthPrime program-—a special, subsidized, primary care–based insurance program for the uninsured. HealthPrime is in essence a Medicaid-like program for the low-income but not lowest income uninsured population. The key point here is that HealthPrime will offer coverage that is both easily available and consistently affordable for low-income people so that a universal individual mandate will be workable for the people who qualify for this option.

It might be possible to simply extend Medicaid eligibility up to 200 percent of the federal poverty level. That approach would, however, move a lot of otherwise employed people out of employer-funded coverage into government-funded coverage and would increase the costs of the total program significantly. Also, Medicaid has a very hard time getting enough providers in some geographic areas. We believe HealthPrime would be far more likely to have a significant provider network in every geographic area.

It was our recommendation in the *Health Affairs* article that the new HealthPrime program be administered in every state by the existing state Medicaid program infrastructure. Why is that the operational recommendation? Because it's by far the easiest way to get that job done. A complete and very robust payment and eligibility infrastructure already exists now in our various state Medicaid programs. The whole infrastructure already works. It's been in place for years. Rather than build a whole new set of files, records, enrollment approaches, procedures, forms, processes, and then hire a whole new administrative staff, the easiest, cheapest, and most effective approach would be to use an infrastructure we already have—an infrastructure that already works—and simply expand its use to include administering coverage for the low-income uninsured who don't qualify for Medicaid.

A major benefit of using the existing Medicaid infrastructure is that quite a few of the low-income people who will be HealthPrime enrollees will also periodically spend some time as Medicaid beneficiaries—as their personal, financial, and work status changes from time to time. If Medicaid administrative processes are used, it will be easy to maintain all of those covered people in a fully integrated and melded database. As discussed earlier, a melded database is very useful for both patients and caregivers. As I've noted earlier in the book, data continuity is often very important for good care. As you will see, one major goal of this entire UCN proposal is to create a usable melded database for each state that can be used to facilitate a high level of continuity of care for each patient. Sharing an integrated database with Medicaid would be a nice first step in that direction for HealthPrime members.

Another major benefit of using the Medicaid infrastructure to support HealthPrime enrollees is that we want to give each HealthPrime enrollee real and meaningful choices of health care systems, teams, health plans, and providers. Most state Medicaid programs are set up now to let Medicaid members either simply use the available fee-for-service providers in their community or select a local health plan as their care system of choice. That same range of options—including any local IVs that exist—should be given to all HealthPrime members—allowing for competition among local care systems for HealthPrime patients and giving each HealthPrime member ample choices between both caregivers and health plans. Americans like choices. Universal coverage in America should embody choices. In health care, choices can lead to new levels of competition where caregivers perform more effectively when faced with consumers who are able to individually make other provider or health system selections. In either a well-structured Medicaid marketplace or a HealthPrime marketplace, people will be happier and the market will perform better when real choice exists.

Community Clinics as HealthPrime Providers

The new system of providing coverage for the uninsured needs to have a particularly strong and supportive role in it for existing community clinics and safety net hospitals.

Community clinics and safety net hospitals currently do the heavy lifting for American health care when it comes to providing care to the uninsured. Community clinics in every major metropolitan area and some rural areas focus their efforts today on providing needed care to uninsured and underinsured low-income Americans. The community clinics almost always do an excellent job of being culturally competent, available at the times when care is most needed, and conveniently located in the heart of the exact lower-income communities where a lot of uninsured people live. The work done by community clinics today is often exceptional. That care infrastructure is absolutely necessary today for the lives and health of millions of uninsured Americans.

Those clinics—and the safety net hospitals that also serve the uninsured and who also tend to be located in the low-income areas of our cities—are almost always underfunded. Staffing is a constant challenge. Maintaining their simple and basic existence is a day-to-day struggle for many of those badly needed caregivers and care sites.

The Universal Coverage Now proposal outlined here has a special dual role for those clinics that gives them a flexible double opportunity to serve HealthPrime enrollees, both on a fee-for-service basis and by enrolling HealthPrime members directly in new quasi–health plans as community clinic plan members. Most state Medicaid systems now have the capability of working directly with community clinics on a fee-for-service basis. Adding both HealthPrime members and a clinic-based mini–health plan option should strengthen and help grow the community clinic system.

That dual payment approach is an important concept. Payment to community clinics can be both fee-for-service and set up as a prepaid, capitation program where the clinics receive a preset monthly payment for each enrolled person. For those community clinic patients who choose to be seen through a fee-for-service approach, the HealthPrime payment rate included in the *Health Affairs* article would be calculated at more reasonable Medicare payment levels, rather than the significantly lower Medicaid payment levels those clinics and hospitals typically receive now for their Medicaid patients. For the community clinics and safety net hospitals who choose to be prepaid for their HealthPrime members, each care system would receive a fixed amount of money each month to provide a menu of defined services for their HealthPrime members. The community clinics who choose that option would be in effect small health plans, paid on a per capita basis, or "capitated" for those patients.

The capitation arrangement for each community clinic and safety net hospital needs to be flexibly designed so that the economics reflect the care available from each clinic care site or hospital. Much like the overall market model outlined in Chapter Ten, each community clinic could accept prepayment for the services it provides directly, and it could have a bonus arrangement paid by the HealthPrime program for meeting a series of carefully defined population health performance goals—like measurably reducing asthma crises for the enrolled population they serve. Asthma, diabetes, and heart disease all lend themselves very nicely to direct performance incentives for the basic community clinic caregivers. By having a shared database between HealthPrime and Medicaid and access to communitywide electronic personal health record information for each patient, the clinics will also be able to avoid many current and future care linkage deficiencies and provide better, more consistent, and more effective care to the population they serve.

Disease registries set up in those community clinic settings have a particularly high likelihood of success. Disease registries can be particularly well funded through prepayment approaches because prepayment does include money that can be used to pay for linkages and communications. Remember the problem listed earlier. Linkages tend not to be a billable event in a fee-for-service payment system, so linkages tend to be nonexistent. In a prepaid system, where the provider is prepaid to take total care of the patient, linkages can be budgeted for and used because they make the total cost of care lower and make care quality better.

The new HealthPrime program needs to make similar financial options available to community hospitals in key areas. The safety net hospitals in many cities now have large percentages of uninsured patients who also do not pay their bills. Subsidies for the safety net hospitals come now from a number of sources, with cost shifting at the top of the list. The safety net hospitals also tend to be geographically located in or near our inner cities, in the heart of our uninsured population. When the uninsured all become fully insured, the safety net hospitals will be paid directly for their HealthPrime and other insured patients. The very best model for continuity of care and consistently improving care quality might well be for the safety net hospitals to also actively participate in various ways to take on prepaid HealthPrime members with prenegotiated capitation fees. Ideally, the safety net hospitals would partner with local community clinics and other local caregivers to form functionally integrated care systems that can provide consistent and effective care to local HealthPrime members who choose the local care team as their designated caregivers.

Some assistance will undoubtedly be needed to help start up those new community-based prepaid programs and to help with initial enrollment. Skilled actuaries will need to review the database for each local caregiver and community and work out appropriate cost-sharing capitation amounts and approaches. The positive impact of systematic prepayment on enrolled patients will be major.

Our previously uninsured populations will benefit greatly from better coordinated maternity care, better and more complete, well-linked asthma care, and much better diabetes care. The community clinics and safety net hospitals ought to be strongly supported as a favored approach to providing that care.

Those clinics and hospitals have already done unbelievably good work when faced with a massive load of nonpaying uninsured people. It would be a shame and a crime not to reward that history, record of achievement, and invaluable, in-place skill set by building on that specific infrastructure as a core of America's future health care reform agenda.

Private Health Plans as HealthPrime Providers

Other private health plans in each market should also be invited to participate as HealthPrime capitated providers of care. Consumers should be able to choose between various plans when enrolling in HealthPrime. Again, an ideal marketplace for the consumer would have continuity of care as a major asset, with people able to retain care systems and ensure personal database continuity even if their insurance carrier changes.

In Minnesota, we set up a system where low-income people who enrolled in state-subsidized MinnesotaCare could choose to get their MinnesotaCare coverage from any of several local participating health plans. Each health plan was prepaid by the state for each enrolled MinnesotaCare member. Inside each plan, no one in the care system or patient population was made aware of which health plan members were direct private enrollees and which were taxpayer-subsidized MinnesotaCare members. MinnesotaCare has been a huge success,[22] in large part because it was built on well-proven in-place infrastructure (whenever possible), instead of creating a whole new bureaucracy and administrative process for health plan–like functions.

In putting together the UCN proposal, a key design strategy was to follow the Minnesota model and work whenever possible through in-place systems, processes, cash flows, data flows, and infrastructure wherever they existed, to avoid the time delays, expenses, and learning curves that always come from installing new organizational approaches. So the UCN enrollment process piggybacks on the in-place tax filing process, and the program administration processes for HealthPrime piggybacks on the current Medicaid infrastructure. The piggybacking process uses current health plans, current community clinics, existing safety net hospitals, and in-place local caregivers as the delivery model.

To get the new UCN program up as expeditiously as possible, and to make the program easy to understand, we should also keep each of the needed set-up steps as simple as possible. The default position for all brand new HealthPrime members upon initial enrollment could well be enrollment in a Medicaid look-alike: a state fee-for-service version of HealthPrime. New HealthPrime members receiving care from any caregivers would simply have that caregiver file a claim with the state through the existing Medicaid system. Once a person is enrolled in HealthPrime, they should be given a choice of competing membership options through the various community clinics, safety net hospitals, and participating health plans. That sequence would ensure that a uniform core enrollment approach is set up for everyone, and it would create the base from which people who become HealthPrime eligible can make other care system choices from the various care systems and health plans who chose to participate as pre-paid HealthPrime care systems.

The Power of the Individual Mandate

The individual mandate approach has its own simplicity of message and impact. It clearly says that everyone must have coverage. Coverage is a necessity. Just like the approach used in Switzerland or the Netherlands, this approach also says that people without coverage must get it—and for lower-income people, that coverage will be made either affordable or free.

Some people worry that American employers who offer coverage now will abandon that coverage once their employees are required to have coverage. I believe the exact opposite thought process and employer behavior will happen if this proposal is enacted. Employers will be more likely to offer coverage to their employees when an individual mandate exists. Why? The new mandate should help employers decide that offering coverage to their employees is a really smart thing to do because employee satisfaction will be affected if that happens. Employers would be directly encouraged by the mandate to help each of their employees meet that new individual mandate requirement, and it will be obvious to each employer that they can make their employees very happy by offering employer-based health coverage at affordable rates. Remember, offering health coverage makes employees happy today, with no mandate in place. Employees will be twice as happy when the employer helps them meet the legal mandate. It's a double win.

What happens if the employer chooses not to offer coverage? If the employer does not offer coverage, then higher-income uninsured people who work there would be required to buy their own coverage. That will cause the higher-income employees to want to work for another employer who does directly help them satisfy their mandate.

In any case, if higher-income Americans do not buy their own personal coverage by tax time, a state default plan will be sold to them as part of the tax filing process. People with higher incomes can simply take the high-deductible plan and pay that premium. Higher-income people who want more complete coverage can apply to a full benefit package set up by each state to provide coverage regardless of health status to otherwise uninsurable people. Most states have those pools already, and they need to be available as part of this overall package.

For lower-income Americans, the process needs to be a little more complicated because we need to make coverage affordable and available for people with various levels of incomes. Mandating coverage but not making it affordable would be a cruel, untenable, and ultimately futile endeavor. We need to facilitate easy and affordable enrollment to get everybody covered.

As noted earlier, lower-income Americans would receive either Medicaid coverage or be enrolled in HealthPrime. Various subsidy approaches can be used for the HealthPrime enrollees. This proposal recommends that people with income levels below 200 percent of the federal poverty level would receive HealthPrime free. People between 200 percent and 300 percent of the federal poverty level would pay 50 percent of the cost of HealthPrime. See the federal poverty level chart in Table 11.2 for our sense of what those dollar amounts came to in 2006.

Under this proposal, the government would need to spend some money. The government would entirely fund the expanded Medicaid program, as well as 100 percent of the cost for HealthPrime enrollees below 200 percent of the federal poverty level—and 50 percent of the coverage costs for people between 200 percent and 300 percent of the federal poverty level. All of those subsidies obviously will cost money. Most plans for insuring additional low-income people fail because there is no workable funding source that can come up with enough money to actually make the program vi-

Table 11.2. U.S. Federal Poverty Guidelines, 2006.

Persons in Family or Household	48 Contiguous States and D.C.	Alaska	Hawaii
1	$ 9,800	$12,250	$11,270
2	13,200	16,500	15,180
3	16,600	20,750	19,090
4	20,000	25,000	23,000
5	23,400	29,250	26,910
6	26,800	33,500	30,820
7	30,200	37,750	34,730
8	33,600	42,000	38,640
For each additional person, add:	3,400	4,250	3,910

Source: Federal Register, Jan. 2006, *71*(15), 3848–3849.

able. We decided to deal very directly with that issue. Recommended new funding sources for the government are shown in Table 11.2. It is particularly important for us all to recognize and deal directly with the reality that each of the proposed subsidies cost money and that money needs to be raised by some source. Selecting an actual source of revenue is, I believe, a key policy decision with far-reaching implications and consequences. It's a fundamental decision that needs to be made very well. A plan to do exactly that is spelled out in the next section.

A Chance for Us All to Come Together

The varied array of enrollment processes that would be needed to institute this new program could give us all a wonderful opportunity to come together as a total American community to help people get health coverage. Initiatives to enroll the uninsured could be run though religious organizations, community organizations, service organizations, employers, caregivers, schools, and other governmental agencies—to let people know that everyone is entitled to coverage and to help people understand and get through the initial enrollment process. We could and should do a superb job of reaching out at the point of enrollment to everyone, bringing all Americans together in the common cause of health care and making sure that our ethnic, racial, and cultural disparities in health coverage become unfortunate historical anomalies, rather than cruel and unconscionable current realities.

Part B: The Source of the Money

So where would the money come from to pay for the expanded subsidized coverage programs? That's Part B of the UCN proposal.

As I noted earlier, that is an extremely important issue to resolve. We obviously can't achieve universal coverage without money. That money has to come from some source. A number are possible. Some people favor simply funding universal coverage from the general tax fund—maybe from increasing income taxes or increasing property taxes. That is not the UCN proposal. Why not? Taxes are already too high in both of those areas. The first problem is that no one is ready to raise these taxes.

The second problem with funding HealthPrime and universal coverage from the general tax fund is that there will then be a huge fight every single year in every legislative and congressional budget between the needs of health care funding and the funding needed for schools, streets, prisons, security, government employees' salaries, and every other legitimate expense of every level of the government. If we decide to fund universal coverage from the general fund, we will guarantee underfunding for health care on a regular basis.

We will also guarantee that issues of annual health care funding will become a primarily political battle—a consistent and constant clash of titanic special interests in a perpetual process of extremely competitive power-base maneuvering to extract resources into and from the health care cash flow. Very bright people in health care will spend their time and energy trying to influence the political process rather than spending that same time and energy improving care. Remember, effort follows funding. If financial rewards for health care come from lobbying, then lobbying will be the skill set of health care leaders. If the real financial rewards come from improving asthma care, then those same leaders will improve care for asthmatics. So using the general fund as the revenue source will both create a set of ongoing political stresses and divert health care leadership from the needed task of improving care.

What we also will not have in that volatile and chaotic general fund political environment will be a pure, appropriately isolated and spotlighted policy-based decision-making process focused on health care as a value and a community goal.

My strong sense after looking at all of those issues is that universal health care would best be funded with a separate dedicated tax source—a dependable, highly visible, directly accountable source of funding. For the purposes of this proposal, I am suggesting that we use two such tax sources: a health care sales tax and what I am calling an in-lieu health tax.

Health Care Sales Tax

In Minnesota a decade ago, we wrestled with these complex financing issues and we settled on funding MinnesotaCare with a health care sales tax. Minnesota expanded Medicaid coverage, expanded coverage for kids, and then set up subsidized coverage for low-income people using a new sales tax applied only to the use of health care services.

As I write this chapter, Minnesota now has the lowest level of uninsured people in the country—beating even Hawaii, with its "employer-mandate" approach to expanded health coverage.[23] The health care sales tax has had a remarkably low level of consumer push-back in Minnesota, in part because the tax is very low and in part because people are so used to sales taxes for other purchases that having them also apply to health care isn't that much of a shock.

Whether the approach worked well in Minnesota is not the key point here. The key point here is that a health care sales tax can be set each year in each state at a level that is highly visible, relatively painless, and financially adequate for the task at hand. If a health care sales tax is set up to fund HealthPrime, and if an expanded program for selling guaranteed-issue full benefit coverage gets funded for high-income people with current health problems, then that sales tax can be both visible and accountable to all parties. It can be set each year in the context of a highly visible debate about what has been accomplished over the past year relative to health care coverage expansion and health care reform. The setting of the new tax level for the next year can be done in a way that gives the public full awareness of what the community is spending its health care dollars on—and public reporting of health care results should show the people of each state exactly what those dedicated health care dollars are achieving.

That focused and public debate and discussion about health care policy and funding does not exist today. It doesn't happen in very large part because the database necessary to fuel the discussion about community care performance doesn't exist. That database will exist, however, if Part C of this uninsured coverage proposal is enacted.

In-Lieu Health Tax

Before going to Part C—accountability and performance—let me finish Part B, the funding. I mentioned two dedicated tax sources needed to create universal coverage. The first is the health care sales tax. The second is a new tax to be charged to any employer who does not offer health care coverage for their employees. All employees who offer health coverage to their employees would be exempt from the tax. The vast majority of large employers and many small employers now offer coverage, and they all would be exempt from the tax.

But many employers do not now offer coverage and, sadly, that number is growing.[24] If we really do want the current employers who offer coverage to continue offering coverage—and if we want additional employers to begin to offer coverage—then a special new in-lieu tax charged only to uninsured employers would make some sense. (Many European countries use a payroll tax now.)

We called that approach an "in-lieu" tax in our *Health Affairs* article because fully insured employers will all be paying their fair share of the health care sales tax as part of the expenses of their health coverage plans for their employees. So those insured employers will all be helping to fund coverage for the uninsured by paying their piece of the sales tax. But employers who do not offer benefits to their employees will not be helping to pay any part of that expense. The in-lieu tax makes up for that nonpayment. It evens the playing field for employers who do cover health care for their employees.

That in-lieu tax money from uninsured employers, added to the health care sales tax money described earlier, would, our economic experts agreed, fully subsidize Part A of this proposal. We had actuaries and economists do some work to figure out how high these taxes would need to be to fund this entire proposal. Interestingly, it appears that the combination of a 4 percent health care sales tax and a 4 percent uninsured employer payroll tax would raise enough money to fund full universal health care for the country. In California, with a higher number of uninsured, estimates are that we would need the 4 percent sales tax, but we would also need a 5 percent uninsured employer tax to fully fund the proposal for that state. In some other states with fewer uninsured and lower health care costs, some combination of 3 percent and 4 percent might be workable.

In any case, if this proposal does end the cost shift from the uninsured, the disappearing cost shift amount more than pays for the sales tax subsidy for the employers. The in-lieu tax or health care sales tax—both at about 4 percent—is real money for employers, but it's less than the 8 percent to 12 percent or more of total payroll now paid by many employers for their employees' health care coverage.[25]

The in-lieu tax also helps answer the question asked earlier: Would employers who now offer employee benefit health plans cancel them in favor of HealthPrime if this new approach is enacted?

The in-lieu tax at 4 or 5 percent creates a steady cash expense for those uninsured employers. Carriers will approach the employers and say, "You are already paying 5 percent. Move that to 9 percent and you can cover everyone, with much happier employees and a healthier workforce." If all the UCN proposals go through, employers who don't offer coverage now would have both a financial incentive to offer insurance and an employee morale incentive. If they don't offer insurance, they will still pay a 4 percent in-lieu tax, and they will be forcing their employees into mandated plans—either Medicaid, subsidized HealthPrime, or more likely a high-deductible plan. For the employers who already offer coverage, they will pay about 4 percent less than they pay now (because there will be no cost shift), and their employees will be happier.

Employers who now offer coverage would, I believe, take a very hard look at the full consequences of any possible decision to drop coverage. Most of their employees would not be eligible for either Medicaid or the HealthPrime subsidy. So dropping coverage would not be simply shifting those higher-paid employees easily to a new safety net plan. It would in fact be making those folks purely uninsured. That would not endear those employers to their uninsured employees. To the contrary, employers in a UCN environment would be strongly encouraged by their own employees to retain group coverage or purchase it. The logic is pretty simple. I do believe that if all employees require health coverage due to the new individual mandate, the employer would actually be less likely to drop coverage than ever before. An employer dropping coverage at the same time that their employees are required by law to actually have coverage would be asking both for major morale issues and for major problems competing successfully with other hirers for desirable employees.

This overall UCN approach will, I believe, cause more employers—not fewer—to offer coverage, and the fact that an employer offers coverage will be much more appreciated by the employees in the face of the individual mandate.

The entire chemistry and culture of health care purchasing will be changed in a positive way when everyone is required to buy coverage, and every employer has the ability to help its employees meet that need in the most affordable way by being the vehicle for purchasing the coverage on behalf of the employees. That entire dynamic will be strengthened if the employers select high performing entities offering real care improvement value and real consumer choices as their coverage of choice. The new market model described in Chapter Ten will have even more traction in an environment of universal coverage, because everyone will be in the model and in the new database.

Part C: Keeping Score

That brings us to the scorekeeping portion of the proposal: Part C. As I noted several times earlier in this book, health care in the United States has a remarkable data deficit. We don't have good information to track the performance of various caregivers. We have a horrible set of care linkage deficiencies that happen when multiple caregivers all take care of the same patient and don't coordinate their care. We know beyond a doubt from the RAND studies and a number of other highly credible reports that there is great inconsistency in health care delivery. We know that people with diabetes do not receive half of recommended care. The problem is, without data we absolutely do not know which half of our patients are not receiving that care.

Given the huge amounts of money we spend as a nation on health care, that massive data deficit is almost criminal. It ought to be completely unacceptable. We ought to know every day which needed care practices and procedures people with diabetes are not receiving, and each of those individuals should have that information as well.

The good news is that we will very soon be able to create an initial database that can be used to give us a huge amount of information necessary to track, coordinate, and monitor care. Since the paper medical record is obviously a complete and utter failure as a population-relevant data tool—and since only a relatively few hardy, enterprising, and enlightened providers of care will have their own medical records fully automated in the next couple of years—the short-term answer to performance tracking for care delivery has to be getting some of the key information we need to know about care performance from the database that already naturally exists in our insurance coverage claims payment systems. To repeat myself one more time, the short-term answer, as outlined in Chapters Two, Three, and Four, is to utilize extensively the electronic database available from the claims payment files of the various payers and formatted uniformly in the personal health record data agenda. As I noted earlier, that database now contains only insured people. If we really want to reform care, we need to add the people who are currently uninsured to that database so we can track key elements of caregiver and community performance across our entire population.

Think about what is possible. Every time a person with diabetes receives care today, information about that care is sent by the care provider to whatever insurer or coverage mechanism is relevant to that patient. The patient's diagnosis is already part of the payment process, because insurers decided years ago not to make mistakes like paying for a C-section for a patient who isn't pregnant. Insurers collect specific diagnosis information with every claim.

Each claim also includes whatever procedures were done for each patient. The procedure information is based on a common set of codes already standardized across the health insurance industry—so if a C-section is done, that code is sent by the care provider to the insurance company and it becomes part of the actuarial database for that patient. All providers use the same code for a C-section.

If lab tests are run, the charges for those lab tests are filed as a claim, along with information about the diagnosis associated with the claim.

The actual clinical results of each lab test—the findings and numerical values—are not usually in the insurance company database. Electronic medical records are a better care management tool because EMRs have that kind of data in great detail. Claims-based electronic records record only the fact that an lab test was done, but even that piece of information can be a useful knowledge point for determining whether or not patients are receiving the full level of appropriate care.

So in other words, several levels of information that can be made available from an insurance claims payment system could go a very long way toward filling the huge and unacceptable data deficit that now exists in health care.

As outlined in Chapter Ten about health care purchasing, that data set would need to be standardized across all payers, and every payer would need the ability to transfer that data electronically from PHR to PHR when people change health plans or communities. All of that work needs to be part of the universal coverage data agenda mandated by each state.

Ideally, if a child is treated for asthma in San Diego under the state Medicaid system and then moves to a private plan or to HealthPrime in San Francisco—or Buffalo, New York—the data about the child's diagnosis, prescriptions, episodes of care, and upcoming care needs should flow seamlessly to the new payer and the new caregiver.

In the time before we implement universal coverage, that data flow inevitably will have huge holes in it. Why? Because, as noted earlier, the uninsured are left out. Uninsured people have no insurance claims database. Uninsured people also tend to not have their basic care data transferred well from caregiver to caregiver. Medicaid plans don't do a good job of getting needed data to private plans or caregivers, and vice versa. There are huge tears in today's data fabric—tears that can be remedied simply by the government requiring the use of standardized personal health record data as both a report and a data flow available from all public and private payers. Medicaid, Medicare, and HealthPrime will all need to put their data and the data flow for that process to work optimally. With universal coverage, that health care data fabric can become complete—and can be used by individual patients to check on the completeness of their own care as well as by care systems and buyers to make sure their patients are having their care needs met.

With that complete data set in place, communities will be able to create targeted, high-leverage initiatives on issues like asthma or diabetes—communitywide initiatives to make sure every kid with asthma is getting his medication and also to make sure that someone is checking to see what might be causing the asthma attacks for each child.

Accountability is close to impossible without data. It's a relatively easy community agenda with data. We need to insist on having that data from all public and private payers if we really want to improve the delivery of care.

Remember, one-half percent of the population spends a fourth of all health care dollars. Ten percent of the population spends nearly 70 percent of all health care dollars. And a lot of those dollars are spent on five chronic conditions—conditions that each lend themselves to community initiatives and systematic care improvement if the necessary data about provider performance is available.

So Part C of this proposal is to do exactly that. Make the needed data available. Also, we need to make it confidential.

Patient confidentiality is an absolute necessity. Databases need to be protected. Explicit patient approval must be required to pass individual identifiable patient data on to new caregivers and new care settings. So we need to carefully protect individualized data.

We also need to be sure that the community has necessary access to aggregated data. We need all data—in confidential form—available to the people who will do population health and provider performance studies and analysis. The macrodatabase for each community needs to be intact in order for overall accountability to occur—intact at the macro level and totally confidential at the micro individual level, where patients want confidentiality as their personal choice.

Patients need to be able to each determine and decide who has access to their individual data. That's the needed rule for individual data. We need a different rule for patient-anonymous, aggregated, community-based care data. The overall cumulative database—without patient-specific identification—needs to be a public utility, like the railroad tracks, with a full data flow process that lets real provider performance measurement finally happen. Without that public utility, overall care improvement agendas would be functionally impossible.

Part D: HealthPrime Benefit Designs

That brings us to Part D of this proposal—the actual benefit package that we suggest should be made available as part of HealthPrime.

This proposal does not recommend any specific benefit packages for the coverage purchased by the general population outside of HealthPrime. It's tempting to design an ideal package for everyone, but a better idea is probably to let market forces and medical science impact that design process—with benefit reengineering fed by a continuous improvement thought process and supported by the kinds of data about specific benefit impact that can be made available by a PHR database for employers, customers, and payers.

But for the people who will enroll in the government-subsidized HealthPrime program, we do need to design a benefit package. We actually needed to do that initially so our economists could assign a price to this proposal. The actuaries cannot possibly figure out a total projected cost of new health care benefits for any community until they know what the specific coverage benefits for those new members actually will be. So benefits were designed to be "costed out" to see how many tax dollars were needed to fund the program. Since benefit design does incent both patient and provider behaviors, it made a lot of sense to put together a benefit package that would encourage both patients and caregivers to act in ways that improve health and care.

The suggestion here is that the same benefit package be used for HealthPrime in all states, but it would be just as reasonable to suggest that some variety and experimentation in that regard from state to state could create some learning opportunities about the impact of benefit options on best care and patient behavior that would benefit us all.

There is no way to approximate the costs of variable benefits other than to create ranges, so the *Health Affairs* proposal recommended one basic benefit set: benefits that look a lot like normal employer group benefits, with a couple of exceptions. So what values and strategic considerations did we use to design these proposed benefits, and what benefits did we propose for the pricing process?

Emphasis on Primary Care

In looking at national health insurance models that are used to achieve universal coverage in other countries, one point becomes very clear very quickly. Every other country places a major emphasis on the availability of primary care. In designing universal coverage benefit packages, every country uses a fairly complete primary care benefit set. When the budget decisions are made in each country, primary care tends to be first recipient at the mouth of the financial funnel. Why is that?

I've actually asked ministers of health from half a dozen European single payer systems why primary care is consistently top priority as the foundation for their systems. The answer I get is based in part on a clear understanding by the governments in those countries of the utilization concentration numbers you read in Chapter One of this book. The universal coverage countries also have a real skewing of their care costs. That skewing looks a lot like ours. But the European health policy folks typically reach a slightly different conclusion from that same data. They look at that data from a more political perspective: as elected leaders who want to be reelected. Politics is very aware of majorities. Governments who look at that cost distribution data see that the vast majority of people use only primary care. So they fund primary care relatively well.

The 10 percent of our population who spend 70 percent of the care dollars are receiving secondary care, tertiary care, and so on—not primary care. In the United States, 90 percent of our population spends only 30 percent of our care dollars, and that 30 percent of our care is provided largely by primary care practitioners. How do we deal with that information? We tend to apply most of our cost-sharing benefit design barriers to the primary care part of the care package, thereby providing and incenting less complete primary care. Even for our uninsured populations, we typically have no guaranteed access to primary care, but our laws do clearly mandate access for the uninsured to hospital and high-tech care.

That model would not work in those other countries. Why? Pure politics. From a political perspective, 95 percent of the population in those countries uses only primary care—so in a purely political system, if 95 percent of the voters are happy, that's good for reelection. But if that 95 percent is unhappy—not getting easy access to or full coverage for primary care—then the voters will be unhappy and the next round of elections could well bring new leaders to power.

So leaders in those countries place their budget priorities on primary care.

It's basic electoral politics applied in a very practical way to health care economics. As a result, people in Britain, Canada, and Sweden all have constant, relatively easy access to primary care. There may be some significant wait times in those countries for hospital beds or tertiary care, but those wait times affect only a very small percentage of the voter-patients, because only a very small percentage need tertiary care.

In the United States, where our system designs, capital investments, and infrastructure building decisions are driven more by available revenue streams than political policy, we tend to underpay primary care. Instead, we build a major and very expensive infrastructure around secondary and tertiary care. Insurance tends to pay rich streams of tertiary care claims in full, so that's where the U.S. care money is, and that's where many of our American health care infrastructure investments are being made.

The consequences of that thinking are obvious to everyone who looks at our care delivery priorities in this country. It also explains in part why we have done so poorly as a nation in taking care of our patients with chronic conditions before they get to those final days of highly expensive, high-tech acute care. We do heart surgeries more often than anyone, but we need to, because patients are not getting the kind of coordinated primary care that would prevent chronic heart disease from becoming acute.[26] Our primary care system is not as robust as the National Health Service in England. Our specialty infrastructure dwarfs theirs.

So how does all of that affect our recommendations for the HealthPrime benefit package?

First Solid Dollar–First Visit Benefits

For starters, my sense is that we need to combine the benefit design patterns of all other universal coverage countries with the insights we now have about the cost impact of consistently doing a good and effective job of treating chronic care patients, and we should put in place a HealthPrime benefit package with first solid dollar–first visit benefits. We should want our HealthPrime members to get their prenatal visits and to get their primary care encounters for asthma, diabetes, heart disease, and depression, without financial barriers.

The proposed HealthPrime benefit package that was outlined in the *Health Affairs* article includes some cost sharing even for those first visits, with a $10 copayment for chronic care or prenatal visits and a $20 copayment per visit for all other acute care needs. Community clinics, safety net hospitals, and other prepaid plans should be able to chose to reduce or eliminate those copayments to attract members and better manage care. But a few copayments should be built into the basic plan.

Prescription drugs should be set up on a similar basis, with a $5 to $10 copay for generic acute care drugs, and a $30 copay for brand-name drugs.

Deductible

A major goal of our care system operational approaches for HealthPrime members should be to avoid unneeded hospitalizations. So the benefit package we proposed for the *Health Affairs* article also includes a disappearing deductible that kicks in after each patient has spent $2,000 for primary care and acute care prescriptions. The deductible would not apply to basic prescriptions used by chronic care patients, but it would apply to a hospital stay. The goal of the intermediate deductible benefit plan design is to encourage primary care and discourage hospital stays.

The proposed deductible starts after $2,000 in care has been delivered, and the deductible in the *Health Affairs* article is also set at $2,000—roughly the cost of one-half day in the hospital. That deductible could also be set at $1,000 or below. Or it could be a fifty-fifty cost share, up to $2,000. The point of that benefit design element is to introduce cost sharing at that point in the care process. The therapy-related goal of that midbenefit deductible design is to fully encourage primary and preventive care and to simultaneously set up a financial disincentive for asthma patients or heart patients to skip taking their medications. An asthma patient who ignores her medications and ends up in the emergency room as a result would face a $2,000 deductible if hospitalized. Likewise, a heart attack patient who does not take his cholesterol-reducing drugs would pay a financial out-of-pocket cost for not following primary care best practices.

The goal is to create a financial incentive for each patient to use preventive medicine in order to avoid her congestive heart failure (CHF) crisis. The care system needs a complete front-end tool kit to help each CHF patient achieve that goal. The message to the patient would be: "You have asthma. Take your medication. Use your inhaler. Avoid being hospitalized. Your inhaler is covered. Your office visits are covered. You will, however, need to pay more money if you are hospitalized. If you do have an asthma attack (or heart attack or CHF crisis), you will have to pay half of the cost for the first day in the hospital yourself. So take care of yourself. Do not skip your medications. Stay out of the hospital."

The clear intent of that benefit design is to encourage HealthPrime patients to use primary care and take care of themselves to avoid unnecessary hospitalizations. As noted earlier, other benefit packages set up with the goal of influencing patient behavior have often taken an opposite approach, using instead a $1,000 to $2,000 completely up-front deductible, followed by full coverage. That pure up-front deductible approach perversely discourages highly effective up-front, preventive care and then equally perversely rewards people with full coverage if they end up in the hospital. Again, if we believe in the power of incentives, we need to set them up to incent the specific behavior we do want, not the behavior we don't want.

For HealthPrime patients who need more care, the benefit is fairly complete beyond the deductible. Once the midrange disappearing deductible is met, their coverage would resume with an ongoing 95-5 percent cost share for any other inpatient care received that year. Again, the recommended coverage is still not 100 percent at that point. Why? Again, to maintain an ongoing level of incentive about relative health care costs. The ongoing patient cost-share piece has two possible uses. One is to sensitize the patient about the difference in price between local hospitals, local imaging services, and so forth. The second use is to have ongoing care creating an ongoing expense, so the financial incentive for the patient is to heal rather than continue to receive institutional care.

Flexibility

The UCN proposal is not dependent on the specific benefit elements of this particular benefit set proposal. Alternative benefit packages could be easily inserted. Some people have suggested that a 50 percent temporary copay would make more sense for low-income people than the $2,000 temporary, half-day-in-the-hospital deductible outlined in the *Health Affairs* article. They make a good point. Full coverage is also possible. But it would cost more money. And it would not create the incentive to avoid the unnecessary hospital stay.

The current cost estimates are based on the benefit plan I just described. That exact benefit plan is basically the one the actuaries used to calculate the cost projections that resulted in the calculation for the tax levels. As I noted earlier, funding needs for those benefits and to subsidize the Medicaid expansion and the high-risk pool coverage could all be met by a 4 percent health care sales tax and a 4 percent uninsured employer in-lieu tax. A more complete benefit set, as shown in Tables 11.3 and 11.4 and in the *Health Affairs* article, would simply increase the costs and therefore increase the percentages for the taxes that need to be raised. That's not a bad thing to consider. But even if the benefit plan is enriched, having a cost share amount of some sort that is triggered by noncompliance with preventive care is probably a good concept to retain in some form.

Universal Coverage Now

So that's the basic UCN proposal: universal coverage. An individual mandate. Tax filing as a verification process. A complete electronic health care data set. Subsidized or free coverage for lower-income Americans. A small financial penalty for uninsured employers. A highly visible, totally dedicated, annually debatable health care sales tax as the funding mechanism of choice. Medicaid infrastructure as the operational tool kit.

This plan can be assembled from existing pieces in months, rather than decades. It should be doable in any given state in roughly two years after it is enacted. One way of thinking about this proposal is the phrase "one, two, three, free." If the program is set up in Year 1 with a 5 percent rebasing of health care costs due to the new tax—and if universal coverage ends the 7 to 9 percent cost shift from the uninsured in Year 2—then the two numbers should offset enough in Year 3—and compared to what costs would have been without universal coverage and a continued cost shift, covering everyone would add no third-year expense. Year 3 would essentially be free. The program would have to be implemented very well to make that happen, but it can be done. One, two, three, free.

It's definitely time to bite the bullet on universal coverage for this country. The ethnic, racial, and economic disparities in care that exist now ought to push us all—actually shame us all—into creating universal coverage at the fastest possible speed. And the new opportunity to link universal coverage to real health care

Table 11.3. Estimated Premiums and Subsidies for CalPrime Options.

Plan A: Annual $2,000 Primary Care Benefit		
Provider Reimbursement Rates	*Monthly Premium*	*Subsidies*
Medicare	$70	$3.2 billion
Medicare plus 20%	$75	$3.3 billion
Commercial	$80	$3.5 billion

Plan B: Primary Care + $10,000 Deductible + Catastrophic		
Provider Reimbursement Rates	*Monthly Premium*	*Subsidies*
Medicare	$145	$5.8 billion
Medicare plus 20%	$180	$7.0 billion
Commercial	$215	$8.1 billion

Plan C: Primary Care + $2,000 Deductible + Catastrophic		
Provider Reimbursement Rates	*Monthly Premium*	*Subsidies*
Medicare	$190	$7.4 billion
Medicare plus 20%	$225	$8.4 billion
Commercial	$275	$9.7 billion

Plan D: Full Coverage (no deductible; some copayments)		
Provider Reimbursement Rates	*Monthly Premium*	*Subsidies*
Medicare	$220	$8.3 billion
Medicare plus 20%	$265	$9.4 billion
Commercial	$310	$10.6 billion

Source: Lewin Group and Kaiser Foundation Health Care Plan estimates in G. C. Halvorson, F. J. Crosson, and S. Zatkin. "A Proposal to Cover the Uninsured in California." *Health Affairs*, 2007, *26*(1), w80–w91.

Table 11.4. Estimated Health Care Sales and Payroll Tax Amounts to Finance CalPrime.

Plan A: Annual $2,000 Primary Care Benefit		
Provider Reimbursement Rates	*Health Care Sales Tax (%)*	*Payroll Tax (%)*
Medicare	1.2	2.2
Medicare plus 20%	1.3	2.3
Commercial	1.4	2.4

Plan B: Primary Care + $10,000 Deductible + Catastrophic		
Provider Reimbursement Rates	*Health Care Sales Tax*	*Payroll Tax*
Medicare	2.9	3.9
Medicare plus 20%	3.8	4.9
Commercial	5.0	6.0

Plan C: Primary Care + $2,000 Deductible + Catastrophic		
Provider Reimbursement Rates	*Health Care Sales Tax*	*Payroll Tax*
Medicare	4.0	5.0
Medicare plus 20%	5.1	6.2
Commercial	7.6	8.5

Plan D: Full Coverage		
Provider Reimbursement Rates	*Health Care Sales Tax*	*Payroll Tax*
Medicare	4.9	5.9
Medicare plus 20%	7.1	8.1
Commercial	9.1	10.1

Source: Lewin Group estimates in G. C. Halvorson, F. J. Crosson, and S. Zatkin. "A Proposal to Cover the Uninsured in California." *Health Affairs*, 2007, 26(1), w80–w91.

reform using electronic data about actual care delivery tells us that the time to act is now.

This full set of opportunities did not exist five years ago. We didn't have the potential uniform, electronic PHR data set that is needed as the foundation of reform. We didn't have the science of prevention as clearly defined relative to the key chronic diseases. We didn't have universal provider numbers for all physicians in America. And until very recently the cost shift burden on the private employers was still relatively affordable—and not as much of an inspiration for real reform as these costs are today. Fixing the cost shift can now pay for universal coverage.

The reality of today's work life and careers is that most Americans will change jobs multiple times over their lifetimes. The old system of purely employer-based coverage made more sense when our parents signed up with a single employer for a lifetime career. But today we need a different level of continuity for both care and coverage. We need a care system, a financing system, and a data flow for each person's care that accommodates and expects change. This proposal does exactly that because it is built around the electronic PHR data set that should follow each person from job to job, insurer to insurer. The paycheck and the employer may change. The patient's history of asthma care should stay intact—and guide future care.

This proposal also takes care of people who fall into troughs between jobs. Low-income people without a job simply get subsidized coverage. Higher-income people get guaranteed issue of coverage, with benefits sufficient to protect their life savings from a catastrophic health event. For people in their working years, the UCN provides a safety net that catches everyone and provides coverage that has continuous data relative to care. It also creates a safety net for early retirees. People who want to retire early today often face huge expenses and major difficulties in getting adequate and affordable health insurance. With this Universal Coverage Now plan, early retirees with higher incomes can simply opt into the government-issued catastrophic risk coverage—or can purchase a higher level of benefits from each state's high-risk pool. Those risk pools are made affordable with heavily subsidized premiums that are also funded by the health care sales tax.

Lower-income people who retire early become eligible for HealthPrime or Medicaid coverage.

Changing jobs and retiring early both become easier with this universal coverage in place. That's the safety net that everyone in America gets in exchange for paying the health care sales tax.

Universal Coverage Now. That, in my opinion, should be the primary health care agenda for the country effective immediately.

Every other industrialized country has managed to accomplish that goal. Every other country has designed a plan unique to its culture, environment, economy, and value system. It's time for us to do the same thing here.

12

So What Should We Do Now?

It really is time to reform American health care. Health care costs are exploding. The quality of care is inconsistent and undependable, and in many cases dangerous to patient health. We don't have an overarching data set to let us know where care is being done well and where it's being done badly.

And we have over forty-five million Americans uninsured, with minority Americans far more likely to be uninsured and significantly more likely to receive inadequate care.

Our consciences and our sense of widespread potential economic damage should both be working together to create universal coverage and universal accountability. Within American health care there are now real and obvious opportunities available to us to do exactly that. One percent of the insured population spends more than 35 percent of our health care dollars. We should be able to intervene strategically and effectively to cut those costs by a third or more, while also improving overall care.

It's time for reform. This book proposes that we as a nation extend coverage to all Americans, funded by two dedicated taxes that will be highly visible and completely protected revenue sources.

If universal coverage ends the current cost shift from the uninsured, the program could pay for itself in three years. One, two, three, free. That's a good deal.

It's time to cover everyone. Now.

This book also proposes that we now purchase real health care reform—that major employers should take the lead and hire infrastructure vendors—or IVs—to create a new two-level, highly functional, consumer-focused health care marketplace—a retail level where consumers can make informed choices about individual providers and procedures, and a wholesale level, where volume buyers (employers and the government) hire the IVs to create consistent improvements in population health for people with high-cost chronic conditions. The current health care marketplace requires consumers to make uninformed decisions about both caregivers and care and doesn't reward caregivers in any way for improving the health of their patients. Those two aspects of the current system cripple it as a mechanism for real reform. Both need to be corrected.

The key to creating a new health care marketplace is data—electronic data. Data need to be uniform, transferable, and universal, across all patients and all providers. The only possible quick-start source of that data is the existing claims payer information files—the information about diagnoses, procedures, tests, prescriptions, and costs that exist now in each payer's computer files. That data needs to be standardized so that patients can use it to track their own care. It needs to be standardized and available so that caregivers treating a patient can have needed convenient access to the full medical treatment history and status of the patient.

It needs to be standardized so we can measure across communities whether or not all people with asthma are getting needed care and, equally important, whether each person with asthma is receiving the right care. Data needs to be convenient, complete, and consistent—uniform in definition and transferable from payer to payer as each person changes plans or communities.

Those data need to be completely confidential, carefully protected, and usable at the individual patient level only when authorized by the patient. Patient privacy needs to be protected. Community data integrity also needs to be intact and protected. So all payers and all providers need to be part of the overall health care data aggregation process, combining individual patient privacy rights with community aggregated data availability in a context that protects both.

This is an attainable goal. Health care reform is possible—and could be achieved relatively quickly. We need to start with the requirements for a transferable patient health record database for all payers: government programs, private insurers, self-insured employers, third-party administrators, and any other process that involves paying medical claims. If the payer industry can voluntarily create that data flow, that would be excellent. If a voluntary flow isn't possible, or if the government programs need legislation of some kind to bring them into the private payer data flow, that legislation should be passed.

We need the ability to set up health care improvement programs community by community, with all local providers part of a common diabetes care or diabetes prevention community agenda. As you read earlier, people with diabetes spend roughly 32 percent of all Medicare monies.[1] The number of Americans with diabetes has more than tripled in the past twenty years.[2] We are irresponsible as a nation if we don't adopt a program to reduce that level of increase and provide better care to people with diabetes.

We can do both—once the full PHR data set is in place, community by community.

There really aren't any good alternatives to a conscious strategic health care reform agenda. We can let the status quo continue—at great cost to everyone involved. We can continue to have over forty-five million uninsured at one time or another—with all the personal and societal pain that involves. We can continue to function in a data-free environment, with no sense of relative performance or comparative accountability.

We could simply shift the cost of care more intensely to each patient, putting everyone on a high-deductible plan in order to get people to spend less money on their own care. But the 10 percent of the population who incur 65 percent of our care dollars will then use even fewer preventive services, and the 10 percent will soon spend 75 percent or 80 percent of our total care dollars.

The alternatives are not very attractive. Let's bite the bullet and systematically reform care.

Every industrialized country in the world has found its own unique path to universal coverage. Let's find a pathway that works for America and do it in a way that gives us a better, more efficient, more patient-focused, and more accountable system than the others. Let's go from last place in universal coverage to first place, with a model that meets the needs of each American.

It's also important to recognize that medical science is improving so rapidly that we are on the threshold of a new golden age for care. Imaging technology is doing almost magical diagnostic work. New tests, new technologies, and new procedures all make the medicine of a decade ago look primitive and mechanical. New genetic science will give us both insights and technological advances that will enable us all—often at great expense—to perform a whole new array of medical miracles by treating formerly incurable and even undetectable diseases. Miracles cost money. George Isham and I wrote about that issue in our last book, *Epidemic of Care*.[3] Miracles cost money, and we all want our miracles to happen. We also want them to be equitably distributed. To make that possible, we need a care infrastructure focused on results, empowered by science, and obsessively committed to systematic process improvement. That's our challenge. If we don't deal well with that challenge, we will face an increasingly unaffordable world of wasteful, unfairly distributed care—and we will trigger political backlashes and economic shortfalls that will keep the golden age from dawning. Let's not let that happen.

We can do this right. The time to start is now.

Be well. And if you're not, be careful.

Universal Coverage Now.

Notes

Introduction

1. Kaiser Family Foundation. "Trends and Indicators in the Changing Health Care Marketplace." April 2004. http://www.kff.org/insurance/7031.print-sec3.cfm, Exhibit 3; Families USA. "Paying a Premium: The Increased Cost of Care for the Uninsured." July 2005, Table 2. http://www.familiesusa.org/resources/publications/reports/paying-a-premium.html.
2. Ibid.
3. Families USA. "Paying a Premium: The Increased Cost of Care for the Uninsured." July 2005. http://www.familiesusa.org/resources/publications/reports/paying-a-premium.html, Table 1; U.S. Central Intelligence Agency. "World Factbook: Rank Order—GDP (PPP)." Oct. 2006. https://www.cia.gov/cia/publications/factbook/index.html.
4. Economic Policy Institute. "Minimum Wage: Frequently Asked Questions." Aug. 2006. http://www.epinet.org/content/cfm/issueguides_minwage_minwagefaq.
5. C. Isidore. "Doctor's Orders: GM, UAW Cut Deal." *CNN*, Oct. 17, 2005. http://money.cnn.com/2005/10/17/news/fortune500/gm_wagoner.
6. C. Noon. "Starbucks' Schultz Bemoans Health Care Costs." *Forbes.com*, Sept. 15, 2005. http://www.forbes.com/facesinthenews/2005/09/15/starbucks-healthcare-benefits-cx_cn_0915autofacescan01.html?partner=yahootix.

7. J. A. Rhoades. "The Uninsured in America 1996–2005: Estimates for the U.S. Civilian Noninstitutionalized Population Under Age 65." MEPS Statistical Brief #130. June 2006. Rockville, Md.: Agency for Healthcare Research and Quality. http://www.meps.ahrq.gov/data_files/publications/st130/stat130.pdf.
8. E. A. McGlynn and others. "The Quality of Health Care Delivered to Adults in the United States." *New England Journal of Medicine*, 2003, *348*(26), 2635–2645. Multiple studies document variations in health care. The Dartmouth Atlas of Health Care, run by John Wennberg at Dartmouth Medical School's Center for Evaluative Studies, has demonstrated glaring variations in how health care is delivered across the United States. For detailed information on health care variations, go to http://www.dartmouthatlas.org.
9. Tom Sackville, chief executive of International Federation of Health Plans, e-mail message to author, Oct. 28, 2006.
10. G. C. Halvorson. *Strong Medicine*. New York: Random House, 1993; G. C. Halvorson and G. J. Isham. *Epidemic of Care: A Call For Safer, Better, and More Accountable Health Care*. San Francisco, Calif.: Jossey-Bass, 2003.

Chapter One

1. Internal Kaiser Permanente data.
2. Agency for Healthcare Research and Quality. "Total Health Services—Mean and Median Expenses per Person with Expense and Distribution of Expenses by Source of Payment: United States, 2002." Dec. 2004 (revised Sept. 2005). http://www.meps.ahrq.gov/mepsweb/data_stats/MEPS_topics.jsp?topicid=5Z-1.
3. U.S. Centers for Disease Control and Prevention. "Chronic Disease Overview." Nov. 2005. http://www.cdc.gov/NCCdphp/overview.htm#2.
4. B. G. Druss and others. "Comparing the National Economic Burden of Five Chronic Conditions." *Health Affairs*, 2001, *20*(6), 233–241.
5. E. A. McGlynn and others. "The Quality of Health Care Delivered to Adults in the United States." *New England Journal of Medicine*, 2003, *348*(26), 2635–2645.
6. Wennberg is the director of the Center for the Evaluative Clinical Sciences (CECS) at Dartmouth Medical School. CECS is a locus

for scientists and clinician-scholars from Dartmouth's medical and graduate schools who conduct cutting-edge research with the goal of measuring, organizing, and improving the health care system. Wennberg's work focuses on accurately describing how medical resources are distributed and used throughout the United States. More information about this effort can be found at http://www.dartmouth.edu/~cecs/about.html.

7. The Institute of Medicine (IOM) is a component of the National Academy of Sciences; its mission is to serve as adviser to the nation to improve health. The IOM's work is organized into seventeen topic areas, including health care and quality, public policy, diseases, and aging. The IOM publishes forty to sixty reports in these areas each year. A complete list of available reports and more information on the IOM can be found at http://www.iom.edu.
8. Institute of Medicine. "Crossing the Quality Chasm: A New Health System for the 21st Century." Washington D.C.: National Academies of Science, 2001.
9. National Cancer Institute. "Cancer Trends Progress Report—2005 Update." http://progressreport.cancer.gov/doc_detail.asp?pid=1&did=2005&chid=25&coid=226&mid=.
10. Agency for Healthcare Research and Quality. "Total Expenses for Conditions by Site of Service: United States, 2002." Dec. 2004. http://www.meps.ahrq.gov/mepsweb/data_stats/MEPS_topics.jsp?topicid=5Z-1.
11. Ibid.
12. Central Intelligence Agency. "The World Factbook: Rank Order—Infant Mortality Rate." Nov. 2006. https://www.cia.gov/publications/factbook/rankorder/209/rank.html; Department of Health and Human Services. "Fact Sheet: Preventing Infant Mortality." Jan. 2006. http://www.hhs.gov/news/factsheet/infant.html.
13. Organisation for Economic Co-operation and Development. "Health: Expenditure and Resources 2006." http://www.oecd.org/dataoecd/7/44/35530027.xls.
14. Centers for Disease Control and Prevention. "Preventing Chronic Diseases: Investing Wisely in Health—Preventing Diabetes and Its Complications." July 2005. http://www.cdc.gov/nccdphp/publications/factsheets/Prevention/pdf/diabetes.pdf.

15. M. de Lorgetil and others. "Mediterranean Diet, Traditional Risk Factors, and the Rate of Cardiovascular Complications After Myocardial Infarction: Final Report of the Lyon Diet Heart Study." *Circulation*, 1999, 99(6), 779–785.
16. J. R. Jowers and others. "Disease Management Program Improves Asthma Outcomes." *American Journal of Managed Care*, 2000, 6, 585–592; T. A. Lieu and others. "Outpatient Management Practices Associated with Reduced Risk of Pediatric Asthma Hospitalization and Emergency Department Visits." *Pediatrics*, 1997, *100*(3), 334–341.
17. One apparent solution would be to ask patients to keep their own records, but that would lead to numerous other problems and is not recommended.
18. See note 6.
19. Partnership for Solutions. "Physician Concerns: Caring for People with Chronic Conditions." May 2002. Baltimore, Md.: Robert Wood Johnson Foundation and Johns Hopkins University. http://www.partnershipforsolutions.org.
20. R. Kuttner. "Everything for Sale: The Virtues and Limits of Markets." Chicago, Ill.: University of Chicago Press, 1999.
21. Centers for Medicare and Medicaid Services. "HCPCS Release and Code Sets Overview." http://www.cms.hhs.gov/HCPCSReleaseCodeSets/01_Overview.asp#TopOfPage.; American Medical Association. "CPT (Current Procedural Terminology)." http://www.ama-assn.org/ama/pub/category/3113.html.; "Relative Value Units and Related Information Used for Medicare Billing." Federal Register, Nov. 15, 2004, 69(219), 66235–66915.
22. Some pay-for-performance programs are being piloted to look at rewarding those levels of performance results. The Robert Wood Johnson Foundation reported on a three-year effort to test seven different pay-for-performance programs; for more information, go to http://www.leapfroggroup.org/RewardingResults/index.htm. However, so far, pay-for-performance initiatives are few and not sufficiently tested.
23. G. Pappas, W. C. Hadden, L. J. Kozak, and G. F. Fisher. "Potentially Avoidable Hospitalizations: Inequalities in Rates Between U.S. Socioeconomic Groups." *American Journal of Public Health*, 1997, 87, 811–816.

24. Commonwealth of Pennsylvania, Pennsylvania Health Care Cost Containment Council. "PHC4 FYI: The Growth in Diagnostic Imaging Utilization." 2006. http://www.phc4.org/reports/fyi/fyi27.htm.
25. Dartmouth Medical School, Center for the Evaluative Clinical Sciences. "A Dartmouth Atlas Project Topic Brief: Effective Care." http://www.dartmouthatlas.org/topics/effective_care.pdf.; Dartmouth Medical School, Center for the Evaluative Clinical Sciences. "The Care of Patients with Severe Chronic Illness: An Online Report on the Medicare Program by the Dartmouth Atlas Project." 2006. http://www.dartmouthatlas.org/atlases/2006_Chronic_Care_Atlas/pdf.
26. National Committee for Quality Assurance. "The State of Health Care Quality 2005: Industry Trends and Analysis." Washington, D.C.: National Committee for Quality Assurance, 2006.
27. G. C. Halvorson and G. J. Isham. *Epidemic of Care*. San Francisco, Calif.: Jossey-Bass, 2003; G. C. Halvorson, F. J. Crosson, and S. Zatkin. "A Proposal to Cover the Uninsured in California." *Health Affairs*, 2007, *26*(1), w80–w91; G. C. Halvorson. *Strong Medicine*. New York: Random House, 1993.
28. For instance, evidence-based care guidelines are in place throughout Kaiser Permanente for major chronic conditions such as asthma, cancer, cardiovascular disease, chronic pain, diabetes, depression, and obesity. Regular measurement activities identify where there's room for improvement in providing evidence-based care.
29. C. Kane. "Physician Marketplace Report, 2001." Chicago, Ill.: American Medical Association, 2002.
30. John Sakowski, e-mail message to author, Oct. 30, 2006.
31. P. J. O'Connor and others. "Mechanism of Action and Impact of a Cystitis Clinical Practice Guideline on Outcomes and Costs of Care in an HMO." *Joint Commission Journal on Quality Improvement*, 1996, *22*(10), 673–682.
32. Medicare Payment Advisory Commission. Transcript of Sept. 7, 2006, public meeting, 132–133. http://www.medpac.gov/public_meetings/transcripts/0906_allcombines_transc.pdf.
33. Ibid.
34. A. Ahovuo-Saloranta and others. "Pit and Fissure Sealants for Preventing Dental Decay in the Permanent Teeth of Children and

Adolescents." *Cochrane Database of Systematic Reviews*, 2004, 3, CD001830.

35. E. D. Beltran-Aguilar and others. "Surveillance for Dental Caries, Dental Sealants, Tooth Retention, Edentulism, and Enamel Flurosis: United States, 1988–1994 and 1999–2002." *Morbidity Mortality Weekly Report*, Aug. 2005, *54*(3), 1–44.
36. M. R. Chassin. "Is Health Care Ready for Six Sigma Quality?" *Milbank Quarterly*, 1998, *76*(4), 510.

Chapter Two

1. The Health Plan Employer Data and Information Set, or HEDIS, is a measurement tool developed by the National Committee for Quality Assurance, an independent nonprofit organization. HEDIS gathers data from health plans about their compliance with best care practice recommendations for a range of acute and chronic conditions. Health plans voluntarily submit data.
2. International Society of Six Sigma Professionals. "Corporate Participants." http://www.isssp.com/?page=corporatesponsors.
3. R. Slater. *Jack Welch and the GE Way: Management Insights and Leadership Secrets of the Legendary CEO*. New York: McGraw-Hill, 1999, p. 225.
4. Robert Wood Johnson Foundation. "Electronic Health Records Still Not Routine Part of Medical Practice, Says New Study," news release, Oct. 11, 2006.
5. C. A. Bond, C. L. Raehl, and T. Franke. "Medication Errors in United States Hospitals." *Pharmacotherapy*, 2001, *21*(9), 1026–1036.
6. C. A. Bond and C. L. Raehl. "Adverse Drug Reactions in United States Hospitals." *Pharmacotherapy*, 2006, *26*(5), 601–608.
7. D. S. Budnitz and others. "National Surveillance of Emergency Department Visits for Outpatient Adverse Drug Events." *Journal of the American Medical Association*, 2006, *296*(15), 1858–1866.
8. E. A. McGlynn and others. "The Quality of Health Care Delivered to Adults in the United States." *New England Journal of Medicine*, 2003, *348*(26), 2635–2645.
9. J. Fraley. "In Pursuit of Perfection: IT's Role in Clinical Process Improvement/Medication Safety." Presentation to Healthcare

Information and Management Systems Society, Oct. 2005. http://www.vahimss.org/presentations /presentations.htm.

10. E. W. Ford, N. Menachemi, and M. T. Phillips. "Predicting the Adoption of Electronic Health Records by Physicians: When Will Health Care Be Paperless?" *Journal of the American Medical Informatics Association*, 2006, *13*, 106–112.
11. CPAS team. "Clinical Pharmacy Anticoagulation Service." *Permanente Journal*, 1999, *3*(2), 26–32.
12. P. Crooks. "Managing High-Risk, High-Cost Patients: The Southern California Kaiser Permanente Experience in the Medicare ESRD Demonstration Project." *Permanente Journal*, 2005, 9(2), 93–97.
13. J. G. Elmore and others. "Variability in Radiologists' Interpretations of Mammograms." *New England Journal of Medicine*, 1994, *331*, 1493–1499.
14. M. Moss. "Mammography Team Learns from its Errors." *New York Times*, June 28, 2002.
15. American Cancer Society. "Breast Cancer Facts and Figures, 2003–2004." http://www.cancer.org/docroot/STT/content/STT_1x_Breast_Cancer_Facts__Figures_2003–2004.asp
16. R. H. Miller and others. "The Value of Electronic Health Records in Solo or Small Group Practices." *Health Affairs*, 2005, *24*(5), 1127–1137; D. W. Bates. "Physicians and Ambulatory Electronic Health Records." *Health Affairs*, 2005, *24*(5), 1180–1189.

Chapter Three

1. R. Hillestad and others. "Can Electronic Medical Record Systems Transform Health Care? Potential Health Benefits, Savings, and Costs." *Health Affairs*, 2005, *24*(5), 1103–1117.
2. Centers for Medicare and Medicaid Services. "National Provider Identifier Standard (NPI) Overview." U.S. Department of Health and Human Services. http://www.cms.hhs.gov/NationalProvIdentStand.
3. Manhattan Institute for Policy Research. "Consumer-Driven Health Care: Freeing Providers to Innovate." March 2004. http://www.manhattan-institute.org/html/_hfm-consumer.htm.

4. UNICEF. "Immunization Coverage Table 2004." http://www.childinfo.org/areas/immunization/countrydata.php.
5. Department of Health and Human Services. "Health Insurance Reform: Standards for Electronic Transactions." *Federal Register*, Aug. 17, 2000, *45*, 50312–50372.
6. Agency for Healthcare Research and Quality. "Researchers Identify Features of Primary Care Practice That Enhance the Quality of Pediatric Asthma Care." *Research Activities*, Dec. 2004, *292*. http://www.ahrq.gov/research/dec04.
7. National Jewish Medical and Research Center. "Asthma Outcomes—Disease Management." 2006. http://www.njc.org/health-plans/disease-mgmt/outcomes/index.aspx.
8. American Health Insurance Plans Center for Policy and Research. "An Updated Survey of Health Care Claims Receipt and Processing Times." May 2006. http://www.ahipresearch.org.
9. Health Net. "Quality Assurance Programs." http://www.healthnet.com/portal/medicare/finePrint.do.
10. "Prevalence of Receiving Multiple Preventive-Care Services Among Adults with Diabetes—United States, 2002–2004." *Morbidity and Mortality Weekly Report*, 2005, *54*(44), 1130–1133.
11. W. T. Lester, R. W. Grant, G. O. Barnett, and H. C. Cheuh. "Randomized Controlled Trial of an Informatics-Based Intervention to Increase Statin Prescription for Secondary Prevention of Coronary Disease." *Journal of General Internal Medicine*, 2006, *21*(1), 22.
12. E. A. Balas and S. A. Boren. "Managing Clinical Knowledge for Health Care Improvement." *Yearbook of Medical Informatics*. Bethesda, Md.: National Library of Medicine, 2000, pp. 65–70. Cited in Institute of Medicine, *Crossing the Quality Chasm: A New Health System for the 21st Century.* Washington, D.C.: National Academies of Science, 2001.
13. D. P. Goldman and J. P. Smith. "Socioeconomic Differences in the Adoption of New Medical Technologies." RAND Corporation, May 2006. http://www.rand.org/pubs/reprints/2006/RAND_RP1199.pdf.
14. A. S. Grove. "Efficiency in the Health Care Industries." *Journal of the American Medical Association*, 2005, *294*, 490–492.

15. S. Rodenhuis and others. "High-Dose Chemotherapy with Hematopoietic Stem-Cell Rescue for High-Risk Breast Cancer." *New England Journal of Medicine*, 2003, *349*(1), 7–16; M. S. Tallman and others. "Conventional Adjuvant Chemotherapy with or Without High-Dose Chemotherapy and Autologous Stem-Cell Transplantation in High-Risk Breast Cancer." *New England Journal of Medicine*, 2003, *349*(1), 17–26.
16. Writing Group for the Women's Health Initiative Investigators. "Risks and Benefits of Estrogen Plus Progestin in Healthy Postmenopausal Women." *Journal of the American Medical Association*, 2002, 288(3), 321–333; U.S. Food and Drug Administration. "FDA Announces Withdrawal of Fenfluramine and Dexfenfluramine," news release, Sept. 15, 1997.
17. S. Fox. "Online Health Search 2006." Washington, D.C.: Pew Internet and American Life Project, 2006.
18. S. Anwaruddin and others. "Ischemia-Modified Albumin Improves the Usefulness of Standard Cardiac Biomarkers for the Diagnosis of Myocardial Ischemia in the Emergency Department Setting." *American Journal of Clinical Pathology*, 2005, *123*(1), 140–145.
19. D. M. Berwick. *Escape Fire: Designs for the Future of Health Care*. San Francisco, Calif.: Jossey-Bass, 2004.
20. N. Gibbs and A. Bower. "Q: What Scares Doctors? A: Being the Patient—What Insiders Know About Our Health-Care System That the Rest of Us Need to Learn." *Time*, May 1, 2006.
21. Institute for Healthcare Improvement. "Shifting to a Higher Standard." Nov. 2005. http://www.ihi.org/IHI/Topics/Medical SurgicalCare /MedicalSurgicalCareGeneral /ImprovementStories/ ShiftingtoaHigherStandard.htm.
22. J. DeFontes and S. Surbida. "Preoperative Safety Briefing Project." *Permanente Journal*, 8(2).
23. Institute for Healthcare Improvement. "100K Lives Campaign." http://www.ihi.org/IHI/Programs/Campaign.
24. Ibid.
25. Mayo Clinic. "Quality and Mayo Clinic." http://www.mayoclinic.org/quality.

Chapter Four

1. S. Li and others. "Diabetes Care and Risk of Kidney Disease in Medicare Elderly Patients with Diabetes: An Instrumental Variable Analysis." Paper presented at the U.S. Renal Data System Symposium, American Society of Nephrology, 2005.
2. U.S. Renal Data System. "USRDS 2006 Annual Data Report: Atlas of End-Stage Renal Disease in the United States." Bethesda, Md.: National Institutes of Health, National Institute of Diabetes and Digestive and Kidney Diseases, 2006.
3. Centers for Disease Control and Prevention. "Preventing Diabetes and Its Complications." July 2005. http://www.cdc.gov/nccdphp/publications/factsheets /Prevention/diabetes.htm.
4. D. M. Eddy and L. Schlessinger. "Validation of the Archimedes Diabetes Model." *Diabetes Care*, 2003, *26*(11), 3102–3110; D. M. Eddy and L. Schlessinger. "Archimedes: A Trial-Validated Model of Diabetes." *Diabetes Care*, 2003, *26*(11), 3093–3101.
5. National Heart Lung and Blood Institute. "Heart Failure." July 2006. http://www.nhlbi.nih.gov/health/dci/Diseases/Hf/HF_WhatIs.html.
6. Ibid.
7. National Heart Lung and Blood Institute. "Heart Failure." July 2006. http://www.nhlbi.nih.gov/health/dci/Diseases/Hf/HF_WhoIsAtRisk.html.
8. J. Braunstein and others. "Noncardiac Comorbidity Increases Preventable Hospitalizations and Mortality Among Medicare Beneficiaries with Chronic Heart Failure." *Journal of the American College of Cardiology*, 2003, *42*(7), 1226–1233.
9. R. Hobbs. "Can Heart Failure Be Diagnosed in Primary Care?" *British Medical Journal*, 2000, *321*(7255), 188–189.
10. American Lung Association. "Trends in Asthma Morbidity and Mortality, 2006." July 2006. http://www.lungusa.org/site/pp.asp?c=dvLUK9O0E&b=33347.
11. Care Management Institute. "Asthma: The Right Thing." Oakland, Calif.: Kaiser Permanente, Nov. 2005.
12. Ibid.

13. S. C. Christiansen and B. L. Zuraw. "Serving the Underserved: School-Based Asthma Intervention Programs." *Journal of Asthma*, 2002, 39(6), 463–472.
14. J. Ritter. "Celebs Call Up on MP3 Cell Phones, Tell Teen Asthmatics to Take Medicines." *Chicago Sun-Times*, May 12, 2005.
15. RAND Corporation. "The First National Report Card on Quality of Health Care in America." April 2006. http://www.rand.org/pubs/research_briefs/RB9053–2/index1.html.
16. W. Phipatanakul. "Environmental Factors and Childhood Asthma." *Pediatrics*, 2006, *35*(9), 646–656.
17. American Lung Association. "Controlling Asthma." Oct. 2006. http://www.lungusa.org/site/apps/s/content.asp?c=dvLUK9O0E&b=34706&ct=67487.
18. P. G. Gibson and others. "Self-Management Education and Regular Practitioner Review for Adults with Asthma." *Cochrane Database of Systematic Reviews*, 2000, *2*, CD001117.
19. National Jewish Medical and Research Center. "Asthma Outcomes—Disease Management." 2006. http://www.njc.org/health-plans/disease-mgmt/outcomes/index.aspx.
20. Centers for Disease Control and Prevention. "Prevalence and Incidence of Diabetes Mellitus—United States, 1980–1987." *Morbidity and Mortality Weekly Report*, 1990, 39(45), 809–812.
21. Centers for Disease Control and Prevention. "National Diabetes Fact Sheet, 2005." July 2005. http://www.cdc.gov/diabetes/pubs/pdf/ndfs_2005.pdf.
22. Ibid.
23. D. Grady. "Link Between Diabetes and Alzheimer's Deepens." *New York Times*, July 17, 2006.
24. Direct costs are the costs of providing all needed care for people with diabetes: outpatient, emergency room, and hospital care, as well as all medications. Indirect costs measure the economic impact of diabetes on society as a whole through loss of productive work time and early death. Source for data: National Diabetes Information Clearinghouse. "National Diabetes Statistics." Oct. 2005. Bethesda, Md.: National Institutes of Health.

25. House Appropriations Committee. *Hearing on the Labor, Health and Human Services and Education Bill*. March 29, 2006. http://appropriations.house.gov/_files/CharlesClarkTestimony.pdf.
26. See note 15.
27. Centers for Disease Control and Prevention. "Overweight and Obesity." Sept. 2006. http://www.cdc.gov/nccdphp/dnpa/obesity.
28. NAASO, The Obesity Society. "Your Weight and Diabetes." http://www.naaso.org/information/diabetes_obesity.asp.
29. American Diabetes Association. "How to Prevent or Delay Diabetes." http://www.diabetes.org/diabetes-prevention/how-to-prevent-diabetes.jsp.
30. L. H. Marchand. "The Pima Indians: Pathfinders for Health." Bethesda, Md.: National Institutes of Health, National Institute of Diabetes and Digestive and Kidney Diseases. 2002. http://diabetes.niddk.nih.gov/dm/pubs/pima/obesity/obesity.htm.
31. National Diabetes Information Clearinghouse. "Diabetes Prevention Program." Bethesda, Md.: National Institutes of Health, Aug. 2006.
32. American Diabetes Association. "Access: Diabetes Research." http://www.diabetes.org/patientinform/default.jsp.
33. T. E. Kottke and others. "Attributes of Successful Smoking Cessation Interventions in Clinical Practice: A Meta-Analysis of 42 Controlled Trials." *Journal of the American Medical Association*, 1988, *259*, 2882–2889; Sacerdote, C., and others. "Randomized Controlled Trial: Effect of Nutritional Counseling in General Practice." *International Journal of Epidemiology*, 2006, *35*(2), 409–415; J. Olsen and others. "Cost-Effectiveness of Nutritional Counseling for Obese Patients and Patients at Risk of Ischemic Heart Disease." *International Journal of Technology Assessment in Health Care*, 2005, *21*(2), 194–202.
34. Information about America on the Move is available at http://www.americaonthemove.org.
35. Ibid; Division of Nutrition and Physical Activity, National Center for Chronic Disease Prevention and Health Promotion. "Overweight and Obesity: Obesity Trends: U.S. Obesity Trends 1985–2005." Bethesda, Md.: Centers for Disease Control, 2006.

36. Information about Shape Up America! is available at http://www.shapeup.org.
37. Centers for Disease Control and Prevention. "Preventing Chronic Diseases: Investing Wisely in Health—Preventing Diabetes and its Complications." July 2005. http://www.cdc.gov/nccdphp/publications/factsheets/Prevention/diabetes.htm.
38. Ibid.
39. Ibid.
40. American Heart Association. "Heart Disease and Stroke Statistics–2006 Update: At-a-Glance." http://www.americanheart.org/downloadable/heart/1140534985281Statsupdate06book.pdf.
41. Ibid.
42. Ibid.
43. S. Yusuf and others. "Effect of Potentially Modifiable Risk Factors Associated with Myocardial Infarction in 52 Countries (The INTERHEART Study): Case-Control Study." *Lancet*, 2004, *364*(9438), 937–952.
44. Heart Protection Study Collaborative Group. "MRC/BHF Heart Protection Study of Cholesterol-Lowering with Simvastatin in 5963 People With Diabetes: A Randomised Placebo-Controlled Trial." *Lancet*, 2003, *361*(9374), 2005–2016; The Heart Outcomes Prevention Evaluation Study Investigators. "Effects of an Angiotensin-Converting-Enzyme Inhibitor, Ramipril, on Cardiovascular Events in High-Risk Patients." *New England Journal of Medicine*, 2000, *342*, 145–153.
45. J. R. Dudl and M. Wong. "From Evidence to Outcomes: Implementing Clinically Effective and Cost-Efficient Population-Based Interventions." *The Permanente Journal*, 2005, 9(2), 63–64.
46. N. Pheatt, R. G. Brindis, and E. Levin. "Putting Heart Disease Guidelines into Practice: Kaiser Permanente Leads the Way." *The Permanente Journal*, 2003, *7*(1). http://xnet.kp.org/permanentejournal/winter03/guides.html.
47. D. P. Chapman, G. S. Perry, and T. W. Strine. "The Vital Link Between Chronic Disease and Depressive Disorders." *Preventing Chronic Disease* (serial online), Jan. 2005. http://www.cdc.gov/pcd/issues/2005/jan/toc.htm.

48. Partnership for Solutions. "Depression: Common Comorbidities." May 2004. http://www.partnershipforsolutions.org/statistics/issue_briefs.html.
49. Ibid.
50. C. A. Mancuso, M. G. Peterson, and M. E. Charlson. "Effects of Depressive Symptoms on Health-Related Quality of Life in Asthma Patients." *Journal of General Internal Medicine*, 2000, *15*(5), 344–345.
51. R. J. Anderson, K. J. Freedland, R. E. Clouse, and P. J. Lustman. "The Prevalence of Comorbid Depression in Adults with Diabetes: A Meta-Analysis." *Diabetes Care*, 2001, *24*(6), 1069–1078.
52. R. Rugulies. "Depression as a Predictor for Coronary Heart Disease: A Review and Meta-Analysis." *American Journal of Preventive Medicine*, 2002, *23*(1), 51–61.
53. L. A. Pratt and others. "Depression, Psychotropic Medication, and Risk of Myocardial Infarction. Prospective Data from the Baltimore ECA Follow-Up." *Circulation*, 1996, *94*(12), 123–129.
54. R. C. Ziegelstein and others. "Patients with Depression Are Less Likely to Follow Recommendations to Reduce Cardiac Risk During Recovery from a Myocardial Infarction." *Archives of Internal Medicine*, 2000, *160*(12), 1818–1823.
55. See note 48.
56. W. F. Stewart and others. "Cost of Lost Productive Work Time Among U.S. Workers with Depression." *Journal of the American Medical Association*, 2003, *289*, 3135–3144.
57. American College of Occupational and Environmental Medicine. "Good Treatment for Depression and Anxiety Means Profits for Employers." News release, Nov. 10, 2005.
58. G. E. Simon and others. "Outcomes of 'Inadequate' Antidepressant Treatment." *Journal of General Internal Medicine*, 1995, *10*(12), 663–670.
59. Agency for Healthcare Research and Quality. "Total Health Services—Mean and Median Expenses per Person with Expense and Distribution of Expenses by Source of Payment: United States, 2002." Dec. 2004 (revised Sept. 2005). http://www.meps.ahrq.gov/mepsweb/data_stats/MEPS_topics.jsp?topicid=5Z-1.

60. Ibid.
61. Centers for Disease Control. "Preliminary Births for 2005." 2006. http://www.cdc.gov/nchs/products/pubs/pubd/hestats/prelimbirths 04/prelimbirths04health.htm.
62. U. S. Central Intelligence Agency. "World Factbook: Rank Order—Infant Mortality." Oct. 2006. https://www.cia.gov/publications/fact book/rankorder/2091rank.html.
63. J. Villar, A. M. Gulmezoglu, and M. de Onis. "Nutritional and Antimicrobial Interventions to Prevent Preterm Birth: An Overview of Randomized Controlled Trials." *Obstetrical and Gynecological Survey*, 1998, *53*(9), 575–585; J. M. Dodd, V. Flenady, R. Cincotta, and C. A. Crowther. "Prenatal Administration of Progesterone for Preventing Preterm Birth." *Cochrane Database of Systematic Reviews*, 2006, *1*, CD004947.
64. J. A. Tioseco and others. "Does Gender Affect Neonatal Hyperbilirubinemia in Low-Birth-Weight Infants?" *Pediatric Critical Care Medicine*, 2005, 6(2), 171–174.
65. J. L. Malin and others. "Results of the National Initiative for Cancer Care Quality: How Can We Improve the Quality of Cancer Care in the United States?" *Journal of Clinical Oncology*, 2006, *24*(12), 1966.
66. M. R. Chassin. "Is Health Care Ready for Six Sigma Quality?" *Milbank Quarterly*, 1998, *76*(4), 565–591.
67. "Policy Brief." Princeton, N.J.: Council on Health Care Economics and Policy, July 2004.
68. For an exploration of high-deductible health plans, see *Health Services Research*, 2004, *39*(4), Part 2.
69. Health savings accounts were created by the Medicare Act of 2003, signed by President G. W. Bush on Dec. 8, 2003.
70. J. Hsu and others. "Unintended Consequences of Caps on Medicare Drug Benefits." *New England Journal of Medicine*, 2006, *354*(22), 2349–2359.
71. Ibid.
72. J. R. Sharkey, M. G. Ory, and B. A. Browne. "Determinants of Self-Management Strategies to Reduce Out-of-Pocket Prescription Medication Expense in Homebound Older People." *Journal of the*

American Geriatrics Society, 2005, *53*, 666; D. P. Goldman, G. F. Joyce, and P. Karaca-Mandic. "Varying Pharmacy Benefits with Clinical Status: The Case of Cholesterol-Lowering Therapy." *American Journal of Managed Care*, 2006, *12*, 21–28.

73. Kaiser Commission on Medicaid and the Uninsured. "Health Savings Accounts and High-Deductible Health Plans: Are They an Option for Low-Income Families?" Oct. 2006. Washington, D.C.: Kaiser Family Foundation.

Chapter Five

1. Centers for Medicare and Medicaid Services. "National Provider Identifier Standard (NPI) Overview." U.S. Department of Health and Human Services. http://www.cms.hhs.gov/NationalProvIdent Stand.
2. Department of Health and Human Services. "Health Insurance Reform: Standards for Electronic Transactions." *Federal Register*, Aug. 17, 2000, *65*(160) 50312–50372.
3. The White House. "Promoting Quality and Efficient Health Care in Federal Government Administered or Sponsored Health Care Programs." Executive order, Aug. 22, 2006.
4. J. K. Iglehart. "The Centers for Medicare and Medicaid Services." *New England Journal of Medicine*, 2001, *345*(26), 1920–1924.
5. E. A. McGlynn and others. "The Quality of Health Care Delivered to Adults in the United States." *New England Journal of Medicine*, 2003, *348*(26), 2635–2645. The Dartmouth Atlas of Health Care, run by John Wennberg at Dartmouth Medical School's Center for Evaluative Studies, has demonstrated glaring variations in how health care is delivered across the United States. For detailed information on health care variations, go to http://www.dartmouth atlas.org. Institute of Medicine. *Crossing the Quality Chasm: A New Health System for the 21st Century*. Washington D.C.: National Academies of Science, 2001.
6. T. Zwillich. "Patients Spend from Health Savings Accounts While Uninformed." *Medscape*, Apr. 21, 2005. http://www.medscape.com/viewarticle/503702.
7. Merck & Co., Inc. "Merck Announces Voluntary Worldwide Recall of Vioxx®." News release, Sept. 30, 2004.

8. Writing Group for the Women's Health Initiative Investigators. "Risks and Benefits of Estrogen Plus Progestin in Healthy Postmenopausal Women." *Journal of the American Medical Association*, 2002, *288*(3), 321–333.
9. S. Rodenhuis and others. "High-Dose Chemotherapy with Hematopoietic Stem-Cell Rescue for High-Risk Breast Cancer." *New England Journal of Medicine*, 2003, *349*(1), 7–16; M. S. Tallman and others. "Conventional Adjuvant Chemotherapy with or Without High-Dose Chemotherapy and Autologous Stem-Cell Transplantation in High-Risk Breast Cancer." *New England Journal of Medicine*, 2003, *349*(1), 17–26.
10. C. Isidore. "Doctor's Orders: GM, UAW Cut Deal." *CNN*, Oct. 17, 2005. http://money.cnn.com/2005/10/17/news/fortune 500/gm_wagoner.
11. B. Corbett. "GM Aims to Hold Down Steel Costs." *Ward's Auto World*, July 1, 2003.
12. R. French. "GM, Nation Losing Out to Health Care." *Salt Lake Tribune*, Oct. 28, 2006.
13. Kaiser Family Foundation and Health Research and Educational Trust. "Employer Health Benefits: 2006 Summary of Findings." Sept. 2006. http://www.kff.org/insurance/ehbs092606nr.cfm.
14. Hitwise. "Health and Medical Websites Received Highest Percentage of Visits from Search Engines Last Week." News release, Oct. 17, 2006.
15. E. A. Balas and S. A. Boren. "Managing Clinical Knowledge for Health Care Improvement." *Yearbook of Medical Informatics*. Bethesda, Md.: National Library of Medicine, 2000, pp. 65–70. Cited in Institute of Medicine, *Crossing the Quality Chasm: A New Health System for the 21st Century*. Washington, D.C.: National Academies of Science, 2001.
16. C. Schoen, M. M. Doty, S. R. Collins, and A. L. Holmgren. "Insured but Not Protected: How Many Adults Are Underinsured?" *Health Affairs* web exclusive, June 14, 2005. http://content.healthaffairs.org/cgi/content/abstract/hlthaff.w5.289?ijkey=1hR6oh4Hhh2jc&keytype=ref&siteid=healthaff.
17. Ibid.
18. Ibid.

19. L. E. Bass and L. M. Casper. "Are There Differences in Registration and Voting Behavior Between Naturalized and Native-Born Americans?" Washington, D.C.: U.S. Bureau of the Census, 1999.
20. S. R. Covey. *The Seven Habits of Highly Effective People: Powerful Lessons in Personal Change*. New York: Simon and Schuster, 1989.

Chapter Six

1. National Committee for Quality Assurance. "Making a Difference: Recognizing and Rewarding Excellence." Annual report, 2002.
2. Organisation for Economic Co-operation and Development. "OECD Health Data 2006: Frequently Requested Data." Oct. 10, 2006.
3. Commonwealth of Pennsylvania, Pennsylvania Health Care Cost Containment Council. "PHC4 FYI: The Growth in Diagnostic Imaging Utilization." 2006. http://www.phc4.org/reports/fyi/fyi27.htm.
4. V. Fuhrmans, "Big Health Insurer to Target Scan Tests as Way to Cut Costs." *Wall Street Journal*, Aug. 19, 2004.
5. Ibid; "Medical Imaging in Canada: 2005." Ottawa, Ontario: Canadian Institute for Health Information, 2005.
6. D. Gesensway. "Internal Medicine Programs Maintain a Steady Draw in This Year's Match." *American College of Physicians Observer*. May 2005.
7. Ibid.
8. Alain Enthoven is the Marriner S. Eccles Professor of Public and Private Management emeritus, at Stanford University. Known as the "father of managed competition," he is one of the founders of the Jackson Hole Group, a national think tank on health care policy. He is extensively published, and his most recent contributions to the health care reform debate include A. Enthoven. "Choice in Health Care." *Health Affairs*, 2006, *25*(2); A. C. Enthoven and L. A. Tollen. "Competition in Health Care: It Takes Systems to Pursue Quality and Efficiency." *Health Affairs* web exclusive, 2005; A. C. Enthoven. "Market Forces and Efficient Health Care Systems." *Health Affairs*, 2004, *23*(2); A. C. Enthoven. "Sustaining a Market-Based Healthcare System." *Healthcare Financial Management*

Association, 2004, *58*(7); A. C. Enthoven and B. Talbott. "Stanford University's Experience with Managed Competition." *Health Affairs*, 2004, *23*(6); A.C. Enthoven and L. A. Tollen (eds.). *Toward a 21st Century Health System: The Contributions and Promise of Prepaid Group Practice*. San Francisco: Jossey-Bass, 2004.

9. Deloitte & Touche. "New Trend to Reduce Corporate Health Care Costs: Employers Realizing Savings Through Multi-Pronged Approach." News release, Sept. 26, 2006.
10. Centers for Medicare and Medicaid Services. "Sponsors of Health Care Costs: Businesses, Households, and Governments, 1987–2004." http://www.cms.hhs.gov/NationalHealthExpendData/downloads/bhg06.pdf.
11. K. Downey. "A Heftier Dose to Swallow: Rising Cost of Health Care in U.S. Gives Other Developed Countries an Edge in Keeping Jobs." *Washington Post*, March 6, 2004.
12. C. Fishman. "The Wal-Mart You Don't Know." *Fast Company*, 2003, *77*, 68.
13. Ibid.

Chapter Seven

1. Association for Manufacturing Excellence. "The Purchasing Machine: How the Top Ten Companies Use Best Practices to Manage Their Supply Chains." *Target*, third quarter, 2001, p. 67.
2. For examples of these networks, see R. J. Lagoe and G. P. Westert. "Community Wide Electronic Distribution of Summary Health Care Utilization Data." *BMC Medical Informatics and Decision Making*, 2006, *6*, 17; J. Halamka and others. "Health Care IT Collaboration in Massachusetts: The Experience of Creating Regional Connectivity." *Journal of the American Medical Informatics Association*, 2005, *12*(6), 596–601; M. E. Frisse. "State and Community-Based Efforts to Foster Interoperability: Tennessee's Brand New Data-Sharing Initiative Has Benefited from the Experience of Four Other States." *Health Affairs*, 2005, *24*(5), 1190–1196; C. J. McDonald and others. "The Indiana Network for Patient Care: A Working Local Health Information Infrastructure." *Health Affairs*, 2005, *24*(5), 1214–1220; and others.

3. Reuters. "Online Health Searchers Don't Check Sources." *Boston Globe*, Oct. 30, 2006.
4. R. G. Wagoner. "From Medicaid to Retiree Benefits: How Seniors Impact America's Health Care Costs." Written testimony to the U.S. Senate Special Committee on Aging, July 13, 2006.
5. Small group and individual premiums are calculated differently. In calculating premiums, insurers are allowed to look at individuals' medical histories and may adjust premiums accordingly or exclude certain conditions from coverage for a period of time. National Association of Health Underwriters. "Consumer Guide to Group Health Insurance." 2005. http://www.nahu.org/Consumer/Group Insurance.htm.
6. J. C. Noreika. "Will You Make Money on LASIK?" *EyeNet*, Jan. 2000.
7. M. W. Malley. "The LASIK Rainmakers." *Cataract and Refractive Surgery Today*, July 2004.
8. I. Brat. "A Company's Threat: Quit Smoking or Leave." *Wall Street Journal*, Dec. 20, 2005.
9. National Center for Health Statistics. "Electronic Medical Record Use by Office-Based Physicians: United States, 2005." Oct. 4, 2006. http://www.cdc.gov/nchs/products/pubs/pubd/hestats/electronic/electronic.htm.
10. J. Wennberg. "On the Status of the Prostate Disease Assessment Team." *Health Services Research*, 1990, *25*(5), 709–716; M. J. Barry, A. G. Mulley, Jr., F. J. Fowler, and J. W. Wennberg. "Watchful Waiting Vs. Immediate Transurethral Resection for Symptomatic Prostatism: The Importance of Patients' Preferences." *Journal of the American Medical Association*, 1988, *259*(20), 3010–3017.
11. Department of Health, State of New York. "State Health Department Releases Latest Report on Coronary Artery Bypass Surgery in New York State." News release, Feb. 13, 2001. http://www.health.state.ny.us/press/releases/2001/cabg2001/htm.
12. H. Sax, D. Pittet, and the Swiss-NOSO Network. "Interhospital Differences in Nosocomial Infection Rates: The Importance of Case-Mix Adjustment." *Archives of Internal Medicine*, 2002, *162*(21), 2437–2442.

Chapter Eight

1. Civitas. "The NHS and the NHS Plan—Is the Extra Money Working? A Review of the Evidence in 2006." Aug. 2006. http://www.civitas.org.uk /pdf/NHSBriefAug06.pdf.
2. R. Pear. "AMA to Develop Measure of Quality of Medical Care." *New York Times*, Feb. 21, 2006.
3. Friedman, Thomas L. *The World Is Flat: A Brief History of the 21st Century*. New York: Farrar, Straus, and Giroux, 2005.
4. Buyers Health Care Action Group. "Our History." http://www.bhcag.com.
5. PR Newswire. "National Business Coalition on Health Conference Convenes Health Care Stakeholders to Advance Value Based Purchasing Agenda." Nov. 2, 2006.
6. U.S. Department of Labor, Bureau of Labor Statistics. "Health Care." Dec. 2005. http://stats.bls.gov/oco/cg/cgs035.htm.
7. Illinois Department of Healthcare and Family Services. "Disease Management: Program Benefits to Your Office." http://www.hfs.illinois.gov/dm/overview.htm.
8. L. P. Casolino. "Disease Management and the Organization of Physician Practice." *Journal of the American Medical Association*, 2005, *293*(4), 485–488.
9. P. B. Ginsburg. "Managed Care Backlash: The View from Communities." *Journal of Health Policy, Politics, and Law*, 1999, 18(1).
10. "Health Plans Facing Managed Care Backlash." *Insurance Journal*, May 3, 2004.
11. B. Gruley. "Suppliers Victims of Japan's Keiretsu?" *Ward's Auto World*, June 1990.
12. National Jewish Medical and Research Center. "Asthma Outcomes: Disease Management." 2006. http://www.njc.org/health-plans/disease-mgmt/outcomes/asthma/index.aspx.
13. N. Pheatt, R. G. Brindis, and E. Levin. "Putting Heart Disease Guidelines into Practice: Kaiser Permanente Leads the Way." *The Permanente Journal*, 2003, *7*(1).
14. Centers for Disease Control and Prevention. "Preventing Diabetes and Its Complications." July 2005. http://www.cdc.gov/nccdphp/publications/factsheets /Prevention/diabetes.htm.

Chapter Nine

1. R. Marcelo. "International Economy: India Hopes to Foster Growing Business in 'Medical Tourism.'" *Financial Times*, July 2, 2003.
2. K. V. Nair and others. "Impact of Multi-Tiered Pharmacy Benefits on Attitudes of Plan Members with Chronic Disease States." *Journal of Managed Care Pharmacy*, 2002, 8(6), 477–491.
3. U.S. Department of Labor, Bureau of Labor Statistics. "Tiered Hospital Plans." July 2004. http://www.bls.gove/opub/cwc/cm20030715ar01p1.htm.

Chapter Ten

1. U.S. Department of Health and Human Services, Centers for Medicaid and Medicare Services. "National Health Expenditure Data: Historical." Feb. 2006. http://www.cms.hhs.gov/NationalHealthExpendData.
2. U.S. Central Intelligence Agency. "World Factbook: Rank Order—GDP (PPP)." Oct. 2006. https://www.cia.gov/cia/publications/factbook/index.html.
3. See note 1.
4. Organisation for Economic Co-operation and Development. "OECD Health Data 2006: Frequently Requested Data." Oct. 10, 2006. http://www.oecd.org/document/16/0,2340en_2825_495642_2085200_1_1_1_1,00.html.
5. Kaiser Commission on Medicaid and the Uninsured. "The Uninsured: A Primer." Washington, D.C.: The Henry J. Kaiser Family Foundation, Oct. 2006.
6. C. Schoen, M. M. Doty, S. R. Collins, and A. L. Holmgren. "Insured but Not Protected: How Many Adults Are Underinsured?" *Health Affairs* web exclusive, June 14, 2005. http://content.healthaffairs.org/cgi/content/abstract/hlthaff.w5.289?ijkey=1hR6oh4Hhh2jc&keytype=ref&siteid=healthaff.
7. See note 5.
8. Emergency Medical Treatment and Active Labor Act (EMTALA). U.S. Code, 1986, *42*, §1395dd.

9. U.S. Department of Health and Human Services, Centers for Medicaid and Medicare Services. "National Health Expenditure Data: Historical Highlights." Feb. 2006. http://www.cms.hhs.gov/NationalHealthExpendData/downloads/highlights.pdf.
10. Department of Veterans Affairs, Office of Management. "FY2005 Performance and Accountability Report: Department Overview." Nov. 15, 2005. http://www.va.gov/budget/report.
11. U.S. Department of Health and Human Services, Indian Health Service. "FY2006 Budget Overview." Feb. 2005. http://www.ihs.gov/AdminMngrResources/Budget/FY_2006_Budget_Justification.asp.
12. U.S. Census Bureau. "Compendium of Public Employment: 2002." Sept. 2004. http://www.census.gov/prod/2004pubs/gc023x2.pdf.
13. U.S. Department of Health and Human Services, Centers for Medicaid and Medicare Services. "National Health Expenditure Data: 2004 Summary and Updated Tables." Mar. 2006. http://www.cms.hhs.gov/NationalHealthExpendData/downloads/tables.pdf.
14. Center for Medicare and Medicaid Services. "Sponsors of Health Care Costs: Businesses, Households, and Governments, 1987–2004." 2006. http://www.cms.hhs.gov/NationalHealthExpendData/downloads/bhg06.pdf.
15. *Employer Health Benefits: 2006 Summary of Findings*. Washington, D.C.: The Henry J. Kaiser Family Foundation and Health Research and Educational Trust, 2006.
16. A. Dobson, J. DanVanzo, and N. Sen. "The Cost-Shift Payment 'Hydraulic': Foundation, History, and Implications." *Health Affairs*, 2006, *26*(1), 22–33.
17. A. Sloan. "Global Investor: Why Toyota Is Beating GM." *Newsweek International Edition*, Mar. 13, 2006. http://www.msnbc.msn.com/id/11675834/site/newsweek.
18. B. Corbett. "GM Aims to Hold Down Steel Costs." *Ward's Auto World*, July 1, 2003.
19. C. Noon. "Starbucks' Schultz Bemoans Health Care Costs." *Forbes.com*, Sept. 15, 2005. http://www.forbes.com/facesinthenews/2005/09/15/starbucks-healthcare-benefits-cx_cn_0915autofacescan01.html?partner=yahootix.

20. HealthDecisions.org. "United Benefit Advisors Announces Results of Nation's Largest Health Plan Benchmark Survey." Sept. 2006. http://www.healthdecisions.org/News/default.aspx?doc_id=82760. The average total cost per employee is more than $6,600 per year; employees pay an average of $2,031 for coverage.
21. Under the Medicare and Medicaid Disproportionate Share Program, hospitals that treat a large portion of low-income patients receive supplemental payments. In addition, federally qualified health centers (FQHCs) and FQHC look-alikes providing primary care receive both federal grant money and enhanced Medicare and Medicaid reimbursement.
22. Families USA. "Paying a Premium: The Increased Cost of Care for the Uninsured." July 2005. http://www.familiesusa.org/resources/publications/reports/paying-a-premium.html.
23. PriceWaterhouseCoopers. "Behind the Numbers: 2007 Medical Cost Trends for Employers." Nov. 13, 2006.

Chapter Eleven

1. British Medical Association. "Fees for Part-Time Medical Services." Dec. 2004. http://www.bma.org.uk/ap.nsf/Content/feesparttime med-privatepractice#1.
2. Commonwealth Fund. "Issue Brief: Entrances and Exits: Health Insurance Churning 1998–2000." Sept. 2005.
3. Emergency Medical Treatment and Active Labor Act (EMTALA), U.S. Code, 1986, *42*, §1395dd.
4. Families USA. "Paying a Premium: The Increased Cost of Care for the Uninsured." July 2005. http://www.familiesusa.org/resources/publications/reports/paying-a-premium.html.
5. Families USA. "Paying a Premium: The Increased Cost of Care for the Uninsured," Appendix Table 1. July 2005. http://www.familiesusa.org/resources/publications/reports/paying-a-premium.html.
6. Families USA. "Paying a Premium: The Increased Cost of Care for the Uninsured," Table 2. July 2005. http://www.familiesusa.org/resources/publications/reports/paying-a-premium.html.

7. Institute of Medicine. *Unequal Treatment: Confronting Racial and Ethnic Disparities in Health Care*. Washington, D.C.: National Academies Press, 2003.
8. A good place to start is the Commonwealth Fund's report "Underserved Populations: An Overview," available at http://www.cmwf.org/General/General_show.htm?doc_id=319068.
9. Centers for Disease Control. "Child and Adolescent Mortality by Cause: US/State, 2000–2003." Sept. 2006. http://www.cdc.gov/nchs/health_data_for_all_ages.htm.
10. Centers for Disease Control. "Adult Mortality by Cause: US/State, 1999–2003." Sept. 2006. http://www.cdc.gov/nchs/health_data_for_all_ages.htm.
11. A. N. Trivedi, A. M. Zaslavsky, E. C. Schneider, and J. Z. Ayanian. "Trends in the Quality of Care and Racial Disparities in Medicare Managed Care." *New England Journal of Medicine*, 2005, *353*(7), 692–700.
12. The Commonwealth Fund. "Minority Americans Lag Behind Whites on Nearly Every Measure of Health Care Quality." News release, Mar. 6, 2002.
13. Agency for Healthcare Research and Quality. "AHRQ Issues New Data on the Uninsured." News release, Aug. 9, 2005.
14. California Healthcare Foundation. "Snapshot: California's Uninsured." 2003, p. 15.
15. R. Busse. "Disease Management Programs in Germany's Statutory Health Insurance System." *Health Affairs*, 2004, *23*(3), 56–67.
16. E. Perryman. "PMI Cover and Claims Reach Record Levels." May 26, 2006. http://www.ifaonline.co.uk/public/showPage.html?page=ifa2006_articleimport&tempPageName=330533.
17. S. Cross, A. Loughlin, and G. Orros. "Private Medical Insurance: UK vs. Republic of Ireland." Powerpoint presentation to an actuarial healthcare conference, Warwick, England, Oct. 2003. http://www.actuaries.org.uk/Display_Page.cgi?url=/proceedings/health2003/index.html.
18. College of Family Physicians of Canada. "Media Backgrounder." News release, Nov. 2, 2006.

19. M. D. Rawlins and A. J. Culyer. "National Institute for Clinical Excellence and Its Value Judgments." *British Medical Journal*, 2004, *329*(7459), 224–227.
20. J. Sterngold. "U.S. Seizes State Prison Health Care." *San Francisco Chronicle*, July 1, 2005.
21. G. C. Halvorson, F. J. Crosson, and S. Zatkin. "A Proposal to Cover the Uninsured in California." *Health Affairs*, 2007, *26*(1), w80–w91.
22. B. Bessinger. "Minnesota Could Be First State to Cover All Kids." *Minnesota Medicine*, 2000, *84*.
23. Illinois Hospital Association. "Percent of Total Population Uninsured by State, 1999–2004." Sept. 2005. http://www.ihatoday.org/about/facts/uninsured.htm.
24. Kaiser Commission on Medicaid and the Uninsured. "Issue Brief: Changes in Employee's Health Insurance Coverage, 2001–2005." Oct. 2006. Washington, D.C.: Kaiser Family Foundation.
25. S. Greenberger. "DiMasi Vows Prompt Health Plan Vote." *Boston Globe*, Nov. 3, 2005; F. Hansen. "Intractable Benefit Costs." *Workforce Management*, *20*, July 31, 2006.
26. Agency for Healthcare Research and Quality. "Preventable Hospitalizations: Window into Primary and Preventive Care." *HCUP Fact Book*, no. 5. 2000.

Chapter Twelve

1. House Appropriations Committee. *Hearing on the Labor, Health and Human Services and Education Bill*. Mar. 29, 2006. http://appropriations.house.gov/_files/CharlesClarkTestimony.pdf.
2. Centers for Disease Control and Prevention. "Prevalence and Incidence of Diabetes Mellitus: United States, 1980–1987." *Morbidity and Mortality Weekly Report*, 1990, *39*(45), 809–812.
3. G. C. Halvorson and G. J. Isham. *Epidemic of Care: A Call for Safer, Better, and More Accountable Health Care*. San Francisco: Jossey-Bass, 2003.

Index

D

I

J

K

L

M